Childhood
Asthma

First published in Ireland in 2011 by
Liberties Press
Guinness Enterprise Centre | Taylor's Lane | Dublin 8
T: +353 (1) 415 1224
www.libertiespress.com | E: info@libertiespress.com

Trade enquiries to Gill & Macmillan Distribution
Hume Avenue | Park West | Dublin 12
T: +353 (1) 500 9534 | F: +353 (1) 500 9595
E: sales@gillmacmillan.ie

Distributed in the UK by
Turnaround Publisher Services
Unit 3 | Olympia Trading Estate | Coburg Road | London N22 6TZ
T: +44 (0) 20 8829 3000 | E: orders@turnaround-uk.com

Distributed in the United States by
Dufour Editions | PO Box 7 | Chester Springs | Pennsylvania | 19425

Copyright © Peter Greally, 2011

The author has asserted his moral rights.
ISBN: 978-1-907593-00-0
2 4 6 8 10 9 7 5 3 1
A CIP record for this title is available from the British Library.

Cover Design Ros Murphy
Internal Design by Sin É Design
Printed and bound by CPI Group (UK) Ltd, Croydon, CR0 4YY

This book is sold subject to the condition that it shall not, by way
of trade or otherwise, be lent, resold, hired out or otherwise circulated,
without the publisher's prior consent, in any form other than that in
which it is published and without a similar condition including this
condition being imposed on the subsequent publisher.
No part of this publication may be reproduced or transmitted in any
form or by any means, electronic or mechanical, including
photocopying, recording or storage in any information or retrieval
system, without the prior permission of the publisher in writing.

Childhood Asthma

Your Questions Answered

Peter Greally

LIBERTIES

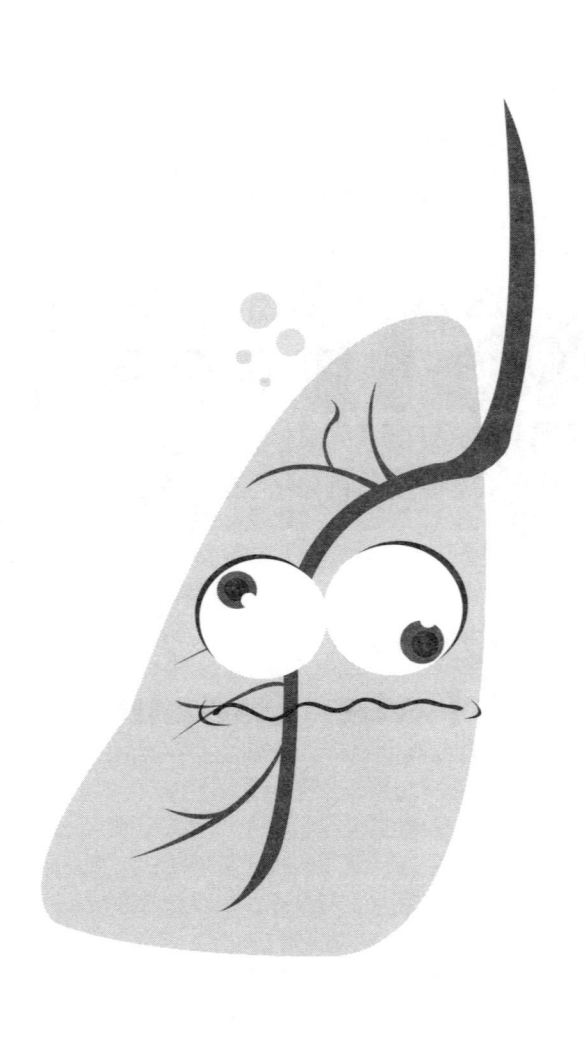

'One must accept
misfortune and mould
it into something good'

Old proverb translated from the Japanese

Dedicated to Cormac Greally

Acknowledgements

There are many people I would like to thank for inspiring and helping me to write this book. If I have omitted anyone, I apologise in advance. Frances Guiney from the Asthma Society of Ireland (ASI) contributed all the scenarios from the asthma helpline. Dr Pat Manning, Chairman of the ASI's Medical Committee, for providing me with up-to-date information regarding the ISAAC studies in Ireland. Thanks to Dr Jean Holohan (CEO of ASI) and Angela Edgehill (Chairman of the Board, ASI) for their encouragement. Special thanks to my consultant colleague Basil, and the respiratory nurses (the two Marys and Catherine) at the National Children's Hospital, from whom I've learnt so much. To my patients and their parents, who bear this chronic condition with great dignity and humour. To my patient wife Rosemary and our children, who put up with my prolonged absences whilst putting this piece together. To my colleagues at the Charlemont clinic (Rita, Patricia, Nikki) who spoil me rotten, and my secretaries Naoimh and Dora, without whose efforts I could not function. Publications like this don't make much commercial sense, so without the support of J. J. O'Connor and Merck, Sharpe and Dome (MSD), who I approached many months ago to contribute to the costs of printing, this book would never have been published. This book is published purely as a reference for patients and MSD had no input whatsoever into its content. Any royalties earned from this first edition will be donated to the Asthma Society of Ireland.

Contents

Six Myths about Asthma   8

In Their Own Words:
Children Describing Asthma   9

Preface   12

Famous Sufferers   16

Your Questions Answered   19

Clinical Scenarios from the
Asthma Society Helpline   129

Further Sources of Information   143

Glossary   145

Six Myths about Asthma:

1. Asthma inhalers cause dependency.

2. Drinking milk makes asthma worse.

3. Asthma is a trivial childhood disease.

4. All children outgrow their asthma.

5. Asthma is only a disease of young people.

6. People with asthma ought to be less physically active.

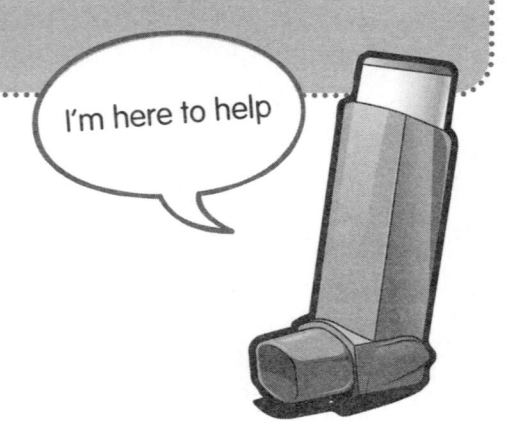

I'm here to help

In Their Own Words: Children Describing Asthma

'Having asthma is like climbing a big, big hill.'

'When you have asthma you can't finish the game.'

'It feels like my voice won't work and my heart is beating too fast. My breathing isn't working, my cough is all chesty and annoying.'

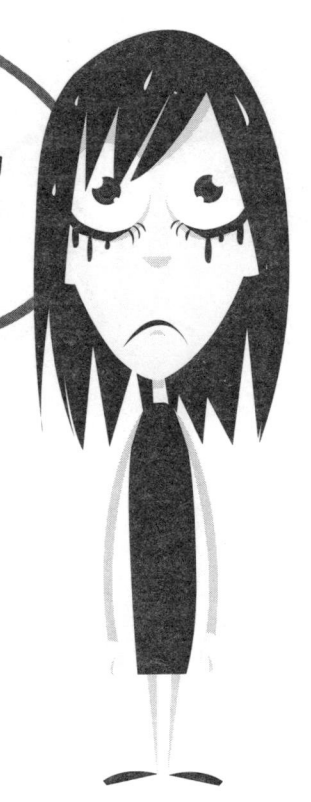

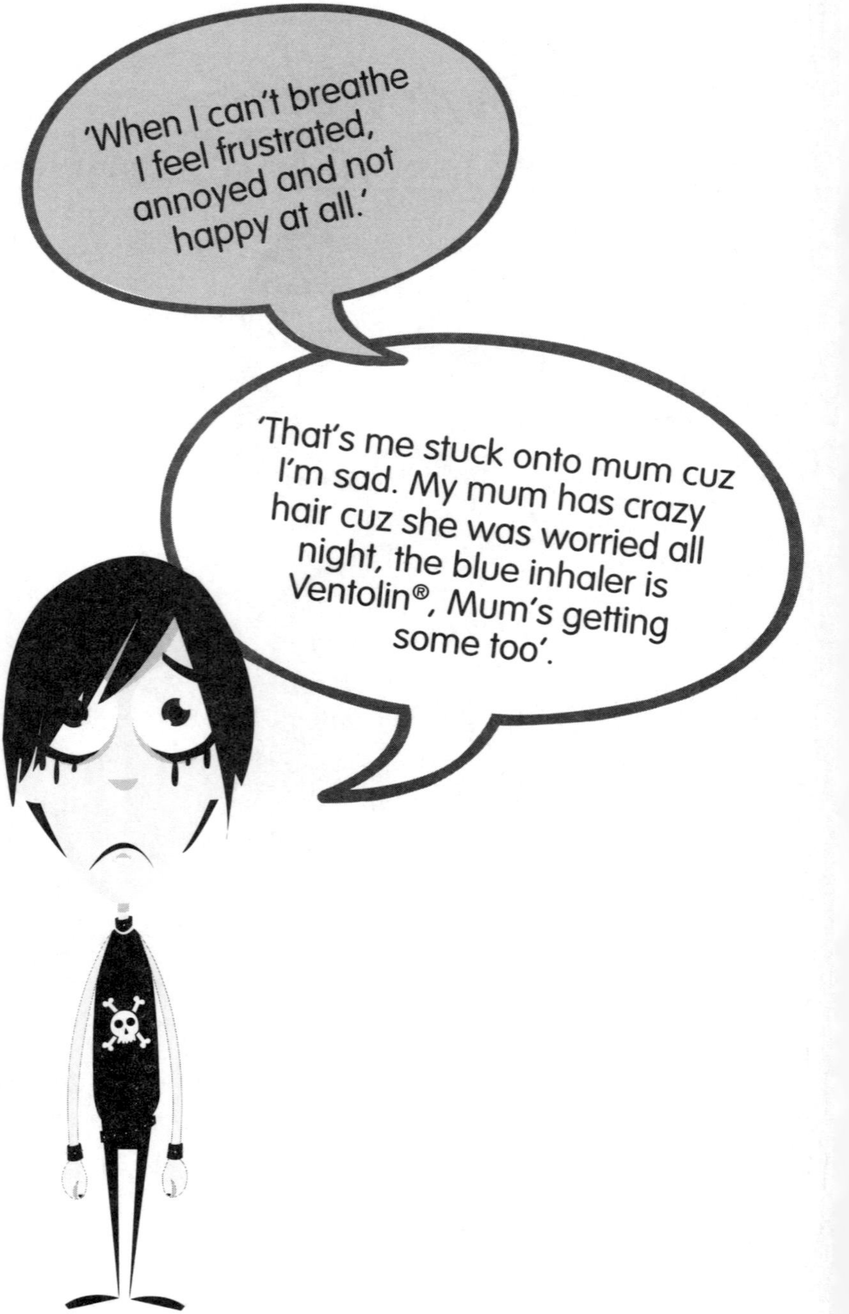
'When I can't breathe I feel frustrated, annoyed and not happy at all.'
'That's me stuck onto mum cuz I'm sad. My mum has crazy hair cuz she was worried all night, the blue inhaler is Ventolin®, Mum's getting some too'.

Caught in a Cloud!

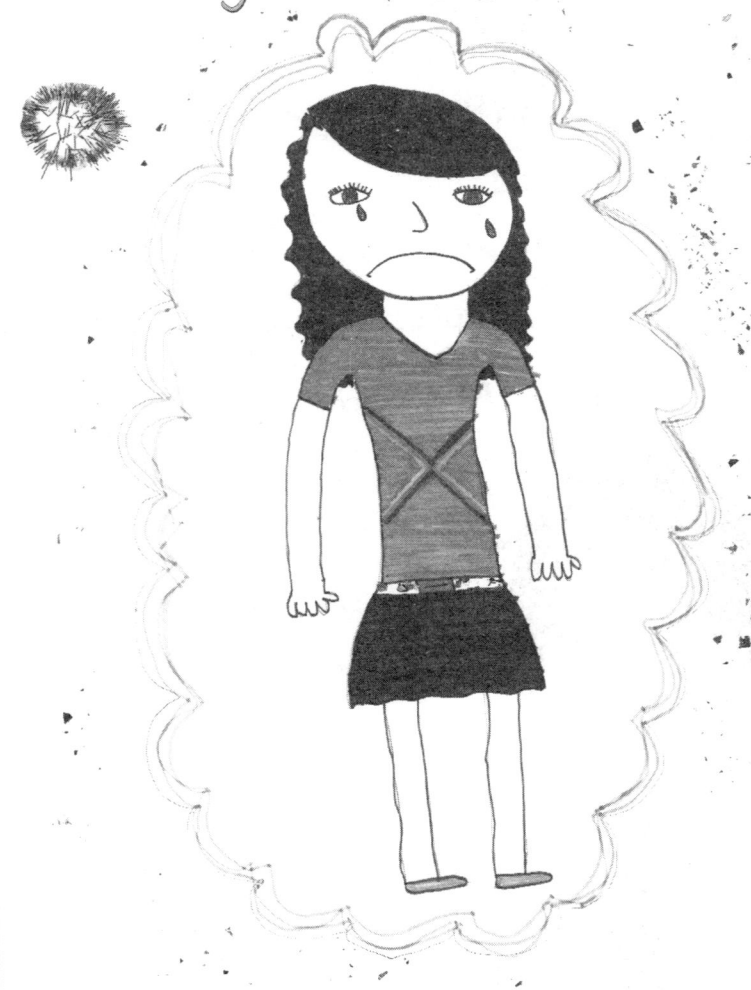

Laura Dolye
Age 12
Winner of Asthma Competition

Preface

Many years ago, when I was eight or nine years old, I would wake in the middle of the night, gasping for air and feeling like I was suffocating. During sport and in PE class, I could not keep up with the other boys in my class. My worried parents brought me to an eminent professor of paediatrics, who proclaimed that my symptoms were due to anxiety. I remember being nursed by my mother, who would advise me to use 'mind over matter' to alleviate my symptoms. At some point, the crisis would pass and I would fall asleep. This pattern continued for two or three years. Eventually, one morning after such an episode, a young, enlightened family doctor saw me, suspected I had asthma, and prescribed an inhaled drug called Intal® (containing sodium cromoglycate and salbutamol). Once I had been started on this, I never looked back. Family mythology suggests that I was one of the first paediatric patients in Ireland to receive this compound. Whether this is true or not, my capacity for exercise improved greatly. In retrospect, it is clear that I had been experiencing exercise-induced asthma symptoms.

> I would wake in the middle of the night gasping for air

I've also suffered from constant nasal congestion from an early age. My blocked nose would get worse during the pollen season; I grew up thinking that everyone had a blocked nose. In fact, I was experiencing symptoms of allergic rhinitis and hay fever. I subsequently discovered that I was allergic to dust mites and grass pollen. Eventually I outgrew my asthma and have since been an active participant in various sports. After the Leaving Certificate, I choose to study medicine at university. It is somewhat ironic that after my internship, where I treated only sick adults, I moved very rapidly into paediatrics, where I encountered children having severe asthma attacks. At the time, I was interested in many specialty areas, including radiology, renal medicine (kidney disease) and respiratory medicine. When it came to choosing a subspecialty, I eventually picked children's respiratory medicine. I subsequently spent two years in research at King's College London, studying the leukotrienes — a class of important mediators of inflammation, allergy and asthma. They were the subject matter of my MD thesis. Little did I think that, within a decade, there would be drugs available for children that would block the effects of the leukotrienes. My project supervisor, Professor John Price, a paediatric respiratory specialist, had trained with the late Professor John Soothill, one of the first allergist-immunologists in the UK. Price approached asthma from an allergy perspective, at the time when most respiratory specialists viewed the specialty of allergy with some degree of scepticism, believing that allergy played very little role in asthma. There was even considerable debate as to the utility of performing allergy tests in asthmatic children. Things have certainly changed since then and we have witnessed an explosion in the number of cases of asthma, rhinitis and food allergy in recent years.

I unconsciously selected a career that involves treating a malady from which I once suffered myself. Perhaps I had harboured a sense of injustice at not having been believed by the first consultant I had seen, who wrongly ascribed my symptoms to psychosomatic causes. Thankfully, most doctors now recognise that although there can be powerful mind-body interactions; the evidence for the inflammatory basis for asthma is undisputed. Thanks to the many drugs that can control asthma, virtually all asthmatic children can now lead normal lives.

There are no signs that the asthma epidemic in children is abating in this country. We will see later in the book that in four successive phases of the questionnaire-based International Study of Asthma and Associated Allergic Conditions (ISAAC) study in Ireland (from 1995-2007), the prevalence of asthma continues to rise. This is in contrast to many developed countries with high prevalence, where rates of asthma are stabilising or even falling. With increased awareness of the condition among the general public and clinicians, and the availability of evidence based treatment guidelines like GINA, SiGN/ BTS or PractALL, it is easy for us to get complacent and one would anticipate improved outcomes for children with asthma. Thankfully, death from childhood asthma remains an uncommon event and undoubtedly there has been a significant fall in the rates of hospitalisation for asthma, particularly in pre-school children. However, these are crude outcome measures.

In 2005 we published results from the Asthma Insights and Reality in Ireland (AIRI study), which randomly surveyed a population of 400 adults and children with asthma to determine their healthcare utilisation, symptom severity, activity limitations and level of asthma control. Over the previous year, 27 percent had either had an emergency visit to the hospital or their general practitioner (GP) and 7 percent were hospitalised for asthma. In terms of asthma control, 19 percent experienced sleep disturbance at least once a week, 29 percent missed work or school and 37 percent of respondents experienced symptoms during physical activity over the previous four-week period. Based on these findings, it was concluded that the level of asthma control and asthma management in Ireland falls well below that of recommended national and international asthma guidelines.

Six years later there would appear to be no significant improvement. In a recent survey of 271 randomly selected children with asthma, it was found that although 92 percent of parents were satisfied or very satisfied with their child's asthma control, 35 percent used their rescue inhaler either daily or weekly. Furthermore, 59 percent experienced night-time awakenings, 25 percent had exercise-limited days and

> **Poor asthma control affects self-esteem**

26 percent missed school on either daily or weekly basis. Poor asthma control affects sleep, school performance, sporting activity and self-esteem. There is an apparent contradiction between parental perception of asthma symptoms and actual control using objective criteria. Parents appear to have a tolerance for symptoms in their offspring and seem unaware of what constitutes good control. So it was for these reasons that I was prompted to write this book. The book is intended to be read on an intermittent basis or as a reference for interested parents and indeed, older children. I have structured it in a conversational, easy to read 'question and answer' style. There may be some overlap in the responses to certain questions and there may seem to be some repetition. However, this was inevitable in a book of this format. This book includes many up-to-date concepts about asthma; however, developments in medicine evolve quickly and some of the ideas discussed in this book will naturally change or become outmoded over the coming years.

Peter Greally, Dublin 2011

Famous sufferers

There have been many famous asthmatics, past and present. These include Beethoven, Che Guevara, Benjamin Disraeli, Marcel Proust, Elizabeth Taylor, Bob Hope, John F. Kennedy and Martin Scorsese. There are even asthmatic sporting heroes, such as Manchester United footballer John O'Shea and Irish rugby internationals Denis Hickie and Ronan O'Gara.

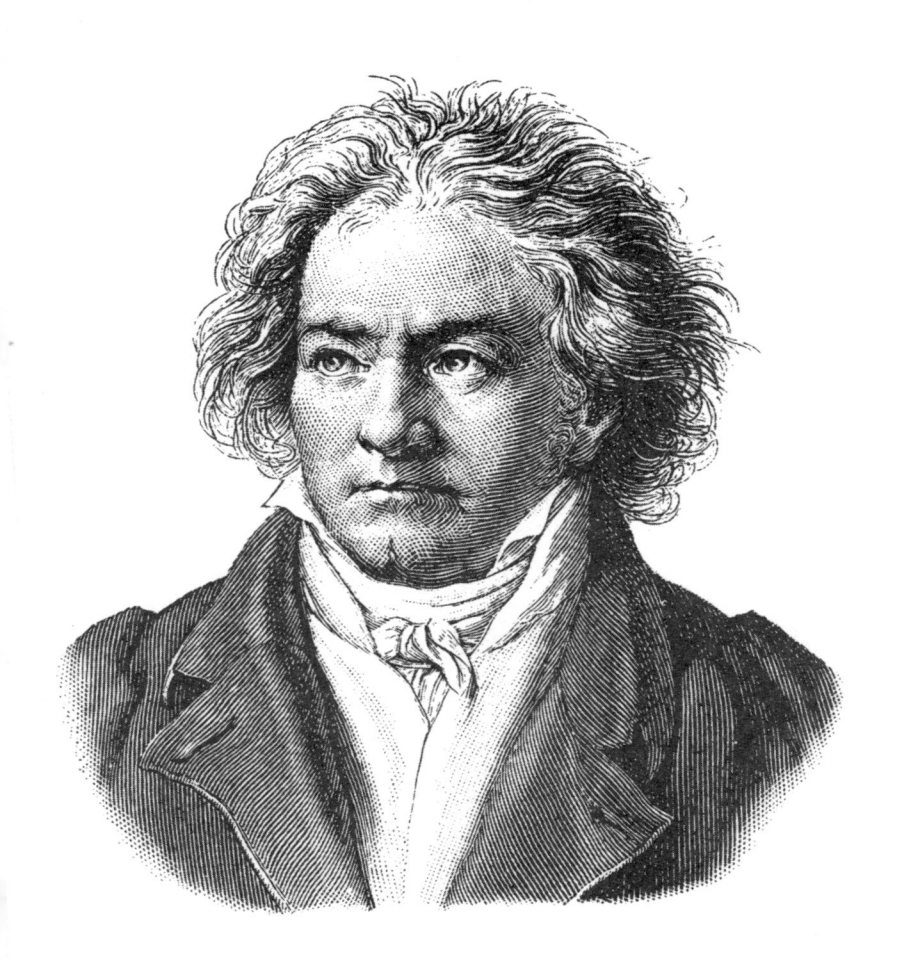

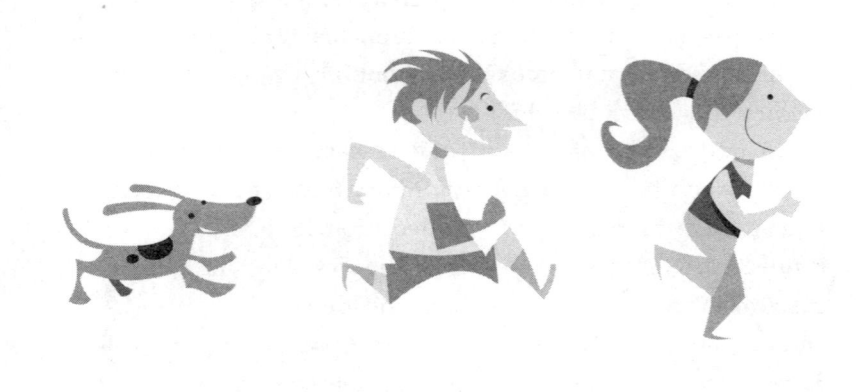

Your Questions

What is asthma?

The word 'asthma' ... from the Greek word *aazein*, ... 'to exhale with an open mouth' or 'to pant'. The condition is characterised by chronic inflammation of the lining of the airways, leading to breathing difficulties due to narrowing of the bronchial tubes. It is common in childhood but may occur throughout life, even presenting for the first time in the elderly.

To understand asthma, it is necessary to understand the structure and function of the respiratory tract. The lungs consist of a series of branching tubes called bronchi, which are connected to air sacs called alveoli. The airways transport gases to and from the alveoli, where the lungs take oxygen and exchange it for carbon dioxide, in a process known as respiration. The respiratory tract actually begins at the nose, which warms and humidifies inhaled air in preparation for its passage down through the larynx (voice box) and trachea (windpipe). In cross section, the bronchial tubes consist of a lining layer (mucosa), which is in direct contact with the inhaled air, and a smooth muscle layer, which surrounds the lining layer.

In asthma, the mucosa becomes inflamed, the lining

the local small blood vessels become engorged, ss of mucus is produced. The surrounding smooth becomes twitchy and irritable, and can constrict the lumen of the airway. The net result is a generalised loss of airway calibre throughout the bronchial tree — a process known as broncho-constriction — which leads to an obstruction to the flow of air into, and especially out of, the lungs. The obstruction is reversible, sometimes spontaneously, and sometimes with the aid of medications. Attacks or episodes of broncho-constriction, or airway narrowing, can be induced by a variety of events, known as trigger factors, which vary from person to person. Inflammation of the airway lining is usually a prerequisite, and predisposes asthma sufferers to symptoms when they encounter these environmental triggers. Bronchial hyper-responsiveness is another important component of the asthma syndrome. If untreated, the airways are more susceptible to broncho-constriction when exposed to specific triggers. The more severe the condition, the more likely it is that the individual will respond to a given stimulus. The degree of this susceptibility to broncho-constriction can be quantified by inhaling histamine or methacholine and taking measurements of lung function in a safely regulated clinical environment; this approach can be used for diagnosis of the condition.

Is asthma curable?

At the time of writing, there is no cure for asthma. However, the condition can be controlled using a combination of environmental measures, trigger avoidance and medications. Nowadays, children with asthma generally live normal, healthy lives. The condition may vary in severity over the course of childhood, and during periods of quiescence, medications may be reduced.

What is inflammation?

Inflammation derives from the Latin word *inflammare* – 'to set on fire'. It is a biological response in which white blood cells respond to harmful stimuli, resulting in changes in the tissue and its blood vessels. The main purpose of inflammation is to remove the injurious stimulus and initiate healing. Infection commonly causes acute inflammation, but not all inflammation is due to infection. Many medical conditions are caused by inflammation that has become unregulated and long-standing (chronic) and is no longer helpful to the body. Examples of chronic inflammatory conditions include rheumatoid arthritis, inflammatory bowel disease, multiple sclerosis and psoriasis.

The inflammation that affects the lining, or mucosa, of bronchial tubes in asthma is frequently allergic in nature and is characterised by cells called eosinophils and mast cells. These cells are the foot soldiers that carry out allergic inflammation. They produce chemicals, like histamine and leukotrienes that produce inflammatory effects and contribute to spasm of the bronchial tubes. In children, asthma is commonly associated with allergies, and can coexist with the other so-called 'atopic' conditions, such as eczema (dermatitis), allergic rhinitis, seasonal rhinitis (hay fever) and food allergy.

What is bronchial hyper-responsiveness?

Bronchial hyper-responsiveness, or BHR, is a key component of asthma, which describes the ease with which a stimulus (exercise, histamine, methacholine or cold air) provokes an asthmatic response in a pulmonary-function test using a bronchial-provocation test. Normal infants are born with increased bronchial responsiveness compared to adults; they appear to lose this responsiveness over time. However, the condition persists in those who develop asthma. Bronchial hyper-responsiveness, although intimately linked to asthma, is not exclusively associated with it, and is observed in other inflammatory airway conditions, including post-pneumonia, bronchiectasis, cystic fibrosis and recurrent croup. Not all children with asthma will have BHR. For example, in those with mild episodic asthma, it may be absent. Anti-inflammatory treatment with inhaled steroids reduces or normalises the degree of bronchial responsiveness in asthmatics.

What is allergy?

Allergy is a common disorder of the immune system and is also referred to as atopy. Atopy derives from the Greek word for 'placelessness' or 'out of place'. Atopy is common in developed countries, where it affects as much as 40 percent of the general population. Allergy is characterised by abnormal physiological responses to normally harmless substances in our environment or our diet; these substances are called allergens. Allergy can complicate inherited immune deficiency syndromes, e.g. Wiskott-Aldrich syndrome, IgA deficiency.

A key component of the definition is the excess levels in the bloodstream of affected individuals of a class of antibody called IgE (Immunoglobulin E), which is attached to mast cells and basophils. On encountering a specific allergen, two molecules of IgE bind to each allergenic piece of protein (epitope), which in turn leads to a chemical reaction within the cell. This causes increased calcium levels that result in the rupture of the mast cell's granules and the release and production of chemicals, like histamine, tryptase and leukotriene, which promote allergic inflammation and broncho-constriction. This is known as a type 1 hyper-sensitivity reaction. Blood IgE levels are high in allergic people but not in normal individuals.

When an allergen is airborne, the reactions tend to affect the nose (rhinitis), the eyes (conjunctivitis) or the lungs (asthma). When the allergen is consumed, it can cause swelling of the lips (angioedema), hives (urticaria), or a serious generalised allergic reaction (anaphylaxis). Anaphylaxis may include the former features, but also has the potential to involve the airway, leading to wheeze and obstruction to the upper airway (stridor) and collapse of the circulation, resulting in low blood pressure. Anaphylaxis can also occur with medications, e.g. aspirin and bee or wasp stings.

In children, asthma is commonly associated with allergies and can coexist with other so-called atopic conditions, such as eczema (dermatitis), allergic rhinitis, seasonal rhinitis-conjunctivitis (hay fever) and food allergy.

Some authorities suggest that there is an 'allergic march', initially presenting with food allergy/sensitisation in infancy, followed by the development of eczema, rhinitis, and later asthma. This pattern does occur in some children, and is reflected in studies which show that, when an individual's allergy status is followed from infancy onwards, the first allergy responses to develop are to foods, and that these tend to resolve with time, only to be replaced with allergies to common airborne or inhaled allergens. Interestingly, infants with eczema may become sensitised to foods that they have previously not ingested, for example egg or peanut. Current theories suggest that this allergic sensitisation may occur through the damaged eczematous skin. Egg allergy in infancy commonly occurs in association with eczema and is highly predictive of later asthma. Peanut allergy can also develop in these individuals.

However, the situation is far more complex than it appears. Research has shown that as much as 40 percent of our population will be atopic (i.e. exhibit a positive response to a commonplace substance on allergy testing). The term for this is sensitisation. However, not everyone who exhibits allergic sensitisation has symptoms: it is quite possible to be sensitised and have no disease. These individuals have been born with, or have developed, a tolerance to a particular allergen. Conversely, at least 20 percent of children with asthma have no evidence of allergy.

What is eczema?

Eczema, or atopic dermatitis, is characterised by a chronic inflammatory and itchy rash disorder, which affects in particular the areas behind the knee and in the elbow creases. It is also known as endogenous eczema, flexural eczema and infantile eczema. It commonly begins in early life and may be followed by the development of the other atopic conditions, such as asthma, food allergy and allergic rhinitis. Approximately 50 percent of asthmatic children will have had eczema. The skin is often very dry and scaly, but may become blistered and weepy. Itching is a common symptom, and scratching can lead to skin infections.

What is allergic rhinitis?

Allergic rhinitis is an allergic inflammation of the nasal airways. It is usually triggered by chronic or repeated exposure to an airborne allergen. It occurs when an individual who has been sensitised inhales an allergen, such as pollen or dust. Adults and teenagers who have long-standing problems with nasal allergy can develop nasal polyps. Seasonal allergy refers to allergic rhinoconjunctivitis occurring in response to outdoor airborne allergens only during specific seasons, e.g. late spring and early summer. Also known as seasonal allergic rhinitis (SAR) or hay fever, the condition is distinguished from perennial allergic rhinitis (PAR), which occurs throughout the year. PAR tends to be associated with regular exposure to indoor allergens such as dust mites, animal dander and moulds. Other causes of PAR include drugs, e.g. aspirin, and occupational exposures, e.g. working in a bakery. There can be overlap between the two conditions: for instance, SAR can occur in 30 percent of subjects with chronic rhinitis.

Allergic rhinitis is a clinically defined symptomatic disorder of the nose induced following aero-allergen exposure caused by IgE-mediated inflammation of the mucus membranes of the nose;

the conjunctivae are affected in 70 percent of cases of SAR. The respiratory tract is a united airway starting at the nose and finishing with the alveoli: inflammation affecting the nose can lead to sympathetic changes in the lower airways, and vice versa. Nasal allergy may be complicated by bronchial hyper-responsiveness and asthma, sinusitis, nasal polyps and glue ear. There can be considerable overlap between allergic rhinitis and asthma. One study showed that 58 percent of patients with allergic rhinitis also had asthma. Conversely, the prevalence of allergic rhinitis in asthma can be as high as 85 percent in some studies. Patients with asthma who deny having nasal allergy symptoms may have inflammatory changes within their nasal mucosa. The pattern of inflammation is similar for both conditions, where eosinophils, mast cells and TH2 helper cells predominate.

What is food allergy?

Food allergy describes symptoms that arise when allergens come into contact with the gastro-intestinal tract (mouth, gullet, stomach or bowels). The first manifestation of food allergy is in early infancy, when babies receive cow's-milk formula. Infants with milk allergy may writhe in pain and arch during feeds. Sometimes they can be difficult to feed, and may be slow to gain weight. Some infants get colic following feeds, but it must be stressed that the majority of cases of infant colic are not caused by milk allergy. Vomiting suggests that the stomach and oesophagus are affected, whereas diarrhoea and bloody bowel movements are suggestive of bowel involvement. Milk allergy in infants may be associated with gastro-oesopheal reflux. Some parents will notice that certain foods or colourants can make their child's eczema worse.

Allergy reactions may be caused by food, preservatives, colourants and drugs. The common foods associated with allergic reactions include milk, eggs, nuts, kiwi fruit and shellfish. The prevalence depends on the food in question, age and the geographic location. For example peanut allergy prevalence is common in Europe and the USA with a rate of 1.5 percent of children, however it is rare in Israel. Hen's egg and milk allergy are also very common with prevalence of approximately 1.6 percent and 2.2 percent of children respectively. Shellfish allergy is more common in adults (2.5 percent) compared to children (0.2 percent). Most children will outgrow egg and milk allergy, whereas only 20 percent will outgrow peanut allergy.

More dramatic food-allergy symptoms include facial, lip or eyelid swelling (angioedema), generalised redness of the skin, urticaria (hives) or itching. Sometimes older children will complain of tingling or discomfort in the mouth following the ingestion of certain fruits, nuts or vegetables. This is known as oral allergy syndrome. This is commonly caused by cross reactivity between proteins in birch pollen, hazelnut and fruits such as apple.

The term 'anaphylaxis' is used for a rapidly progressive, severe reaction, which affects multiple systems within the body and can lead to shock and may cause death. It includes respiratory symptoms such as stridor, choking cough, wheezing, laboured breathing, and blueness of the lips and tongue (cyanosis). Sweating and collapse are caused by low blood pressure. The onset is often rapid, and the episode can be aborted by an adrenalin injection. Children who suffer from asthma and food allergy invariably require access to an adrenalin pen, because any accidental exposure to the allergen has the potential to provoke severe respiratory symptoms.

Do asthma and allergic disorders run in families?

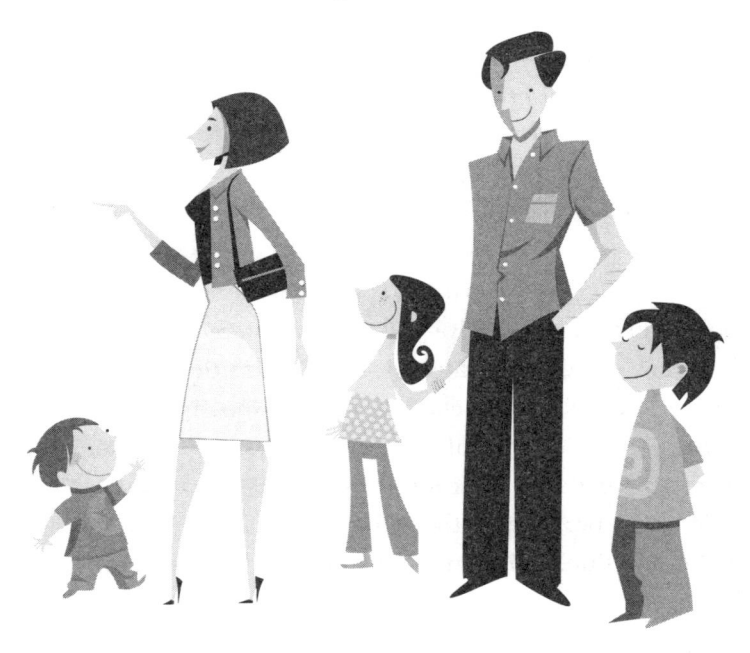

Often there can be a significant hereditary component to these diseases, and family histories can be strongly influential in this group of disorders. A maternal history of asthma has been consistently shown to be more predictive of the development of asthma than a paternal history. In childhood, asthma is more common in boys. This gender bias reverses in adulthood, where women are more frequently affected. The Asthma Prediction Index was derived from the Tucson Birth Cohort, where 1,200 randomly selected infants were followed for nearly thirty years. Children were characterised in terms of their family history of asthma and co-existing allergy diseases. Symptoms, lung function and allergy status were assessed at regular intervals. The infants have now grown into mature adults, and the information gathered has helped doctors identify patterns of illness. The index is comprised of two major criteria (parental asthma and personal history of eczema) and three minor criteria (wheeze outside of head colds, allergic rhinitis and increased blood eosinophils). If a child aged two to three years had one major or two minor criteria, then the odds of them having asthma at age six to eleven years were very high in children who had frequently wheezed in the previous year.

> **Are asthma and allergies diseases of the twentieth and twenty-first centuries?**

Asthma is far from being a recent condition. It was described in the famous Eber Papyrus from ancient Egypt. In circa 450 BC, Hippocrates described the episodic nature of the attacks and observed that they were triggered by moisture and changes in the weather. He also observed a relationship between asthma and certain occupations, noting that fishermen, tailors and metal workers were prone to the disorder. In 1190 AD, the first book on asthma was written, by a Jewish physician, Moses Maimounides, who treated the son of the Sultan Saladin for asthma and melancholia. This is widely believed to be the first description of the psychosomatic component of asthma.

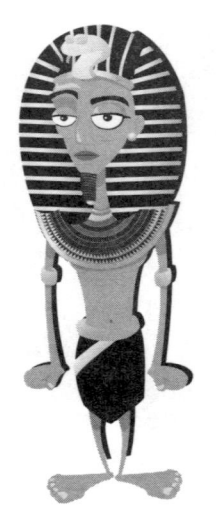

Physicians in the seventeenth and eighteenth centuries recognised the constriction of the bronchial tubes and coined the term 'epilepsy of the lungs'. Sir John Floyer, a physician from Lichfield, who had suffered from asthma for more than sixty years, recognised the curative properties of caffeine. He recommended liberal consumption of coffee, noting its beneficial effect on his breathing. It is now known that the group of asthma medications called methylxanthines are derived from caffeine.

Allergies are not a new phenomenon either. One of the earliest descriptions of anaphlaxis (severe allergic reaction) comes from Egypt, where in 3640 BC King Menses died shortly after having been stung by a wasp. There are descriptions from Roman times when Britannicus, the son of the Emperor Claudius, developed acute rhinitis symptoms on exposure to his horse. The first systematic description of hay fever was in 1819, by Dr John Bostock. The first skin test was performed by Dr Charles Blakely in 1869. While investigating his own hay fever, Dr Blakely introduced grass pollen into the skin via an abrasion, to cause a weal.

What are the symptoms of asthma?

Not all children with asthma will have the same symptoms. There can often be a preceding viral illness, with snuffles or cold-like symptoms. Symptoms will depend on your child's age: for example, infants and toddlers won't complain of exercise-related breathlessness, but will simply do less. The symptoms of asthma can reflect the underlying pathophysiology. Wheeze is the dominant symptom of asthma, but not all wheeze is due to asthma, and similarly, not every asthmatic wheezes. Wheeze is a whistling sound that occurs during exhalation; it is caused by airflow through narrowed bronchial tubes. Narrowing of the airway can be caused by conditions other than asthma. Your family doctor will take a careful history and perform a physical examination in order to rule out the other less common possibilities.

> 'All that wheezes is not asthma '
> CHEVALIER JACKSON,
> Laryngologist; *Boston Medical Quarterly*, 1865.

What other conditions may mimic asthma?

Many, much rarer conditions can be associated with narrowing of the airway, and can produce wheeze and cough:

Inhaled foreign body (e.g. peanut.) This often occurs in a pre-school child. A history of choking will be present in only 50 percent of cases. Treatment involves removal of the foreign body by bronchoscopy, under general anaesthetic.

Cystic Fibrosis (CF) is a life-shortening genetic condition of mucus-producing cells throughout the body. It principally affects the lungs, sweat glands and pancreas. It may present with cough, wheeze and breathlessness, which may be confused with asthma. Children with CF may also have loose stools and be underweight. The condition is diagnosed by sweat test. Newborn screening for CF in Ireland is expected to be introduced in 2011.

Congenital abnormalities of trachea or bronchus such as tracheomalacia or bronchomalacia, where localised weakness of the airway wall leads to floppiness and collapse of the airway leading to wheeze.

Inherited immune deficiency. There are many disorders of the immune system that predispose affected children to respiratory infections and wheeze. The most common type is IgA deficiency, which affects 1 in 600 people; this is often associated with atopy and asthma.

Primary Ciliary Dyskinesia. Cilia are projections that extrude from respiratory cells; their function is to facilitate the clearance of microbes and pollutants from both the upper and lower respiratory tracts. Rarely, in some children these cilia fail to function correctly, and this may result in recurrent upper and lower respiratory tract infection. Primary Ciliary Dyskinesia is treated with chest physiotherapy, and respiratory infection is treated with antibiotics.

Bronchiectasis is a disease state defined by localised, irreversible dilation of part of the bronchial tree. It may be caused by a severe pneumonia, immune deficiency, CF, or ciliary dyskinesia. Bronchiectasis is treated with chest physiotherapy and respiratory infection is treated with antibiotics.

Gastro-oesophageal reflux with aspiration, where the contents of the stomach are passed back into the gullet (because of malfunction of the valve, or sphincter, between stomach and oesophagus) and then inhaled into the respiratory tract.

Direct aspiration via fistula (hole) between trachea and oesophagus. Very rarely, infants can be born with communications between the respiratory tract and the gullet, where formula can pass into the respiratory tract, leading to coughing and wheeze. Symptoms often occur after feeds. Surgical closure of the defect is required.

Vocal cord dysfunction (VCD) is a condition that affects the vocal cords. It is characterised by full or partial vocal fold closure, which usually occurs during inhalation for short periods of time; however, the condition can occur during both inhalation and exhalation. VCD can produce an expiratory sound, which may mimic asthma. The condition is diagnosed at laryngoscopy, and treatment usually consists of speech and language therapy.

Typically, asthma symptoms are worse at night or upon wakening. Pre-school children and toddlers have less wheeze than older children; individuals in this age group may present with recurrent wheezy chest infections. In fact, it is usually viral upper respiratory infections that precede and trigger cough and wheeze. These children often receive multiple courses of antibiotics without major improvement.

One has to be careful about making a diagnosis of asthma in children less than two years. Recurrent respiratory illness with wheeze is common in this age group, and the symptoms can be identical to those of asthma. However, we now know, from longitudinal population studies like the Tucson Children's Birth Cohort, that the majority of these children are non-atopic wheezers, whose symptoms are only triggered by viral upper respiratory infection, and that the condition will subside by school age.

Sometimes wheeze will be associated with chest discomfort or even pain. Pre-school children don't localise pain very well, and in this age group, tummy ache may be a manifestation of asthma. Where cough is a symptom of asthma, it is usually dry, worse at night or on exertion. Cough may be the only symptom of asthma; however, clinicians are more reticent about making a diagnosis using only cough as the basis.

In older children who participate in more formal exercise, it may be noticed that they can't keep up, or that they lack stamina.

Sometimes these children opt for more sedentary pursuits, or, instead of playing midfield, prefer to play in goal, for example. It has been shown using accelerometers (devices which measure the number of footsteps) that asthmatic children are less active than their peers.

Exertional symptoms can reflect poor asthma control, yet exercise symptoms may dominate, and can occur against a background of generally good control. There is a specific form of asthma where exercise is the only trigger; this is termed exercise-induced asthma. Leukotrienes have been specifically implicated in the development of this form of asthma, and treatment using antileukotrienes may be particularly effective.

What are the signs of an asthma attack?

Signs of an asthma attack again depend on your child's age. Respiratory rate varies with age: normal values range from sixty breaths per minute in a newborn, to twelve breaths per minute in an adolescent (see table). Respiratory rates will increase with moderate or severe asthma attacks. In infants and toddlers, parents may notice this breathlessness and a reluctance or inability to feed, an increase in the rate of breathing, or both. They may notice in-drawing (retractions) of the lower chest wall between the ribs and above the sternum (breastbone). If the episode is severe, they may notice a bluish discoloration of the tongue or lips (cyanosis). This is a sign of insufficient oxygen reaching the bloodstream.

Older children will complain of breathing difficulty and may not be able to speak in sentences without gasping for breath. Some children describe an asthma attack as being like trying to breathe in and out through a straw in the mouth. In older children, the increased effort of breathing may manifest itself with an increase in the activity of the neck muscles (the accessory muscles of respiration). If the child is old enough to use a peak flow rate monitor, then it may be possible to take the best of three measurements, which will be reduced compared to their baseline readings, or those predicted for age, sex, race and height.

If your child ends up in an emergency department, pulse oximetry may be performed to measure the amount of oxygen in the bloodstream. This is a simple painless test which involves attaching a probe to the finger, toe or ear lobe. If a child is lacking oxygen, readings will be low. This usually signifies a more severe episode, and oxygen will be administered.

Infants 6 weeks	20-45 breaths per minute
1-4 years	20-35 breaths per minute
5-14 years	15-25 breaths per minute
14-18 years	12-22 breaths per minute

Is all children's asthma the same?

The short answer is no. There are probably different subtypes of asthma. We know that children's asthma may differ greatly between one child and another in terms of symptoms, severity and triggers. Some children may only cough, whilst others will be more prone to wheeze. In approximately 50 percent of cases, children's asthma is mild and episodic; in 40 percent of cases, it is more persistent and moderately severe; and in 5 percent of cases, it is severe. In some children, particularly those of pre-school age, asthma is only triggered by viral upper respiratory tract infections. In others, their symptoms may be triggered by viral illness and allergens. Some asthma is only triggered by exercise.

Is asthma common in Ireland?

In Ireland, in common with other developed countries, the prevalence of asthma has more than quadrupled between the 1980s and 2000. In 1983, a questionnaire was completed by almost three thousand Irish schoolchildren (four to nineteen years); this was repeated again nine years later in the same age group. The questionnaire screened children for asthma-like symptoms, eczema and hay fever. The researchers found that in 1983, asthma prevalence was 4.4 percent, and that over the subsequent decade, the rate had increased to 11.9 percent.

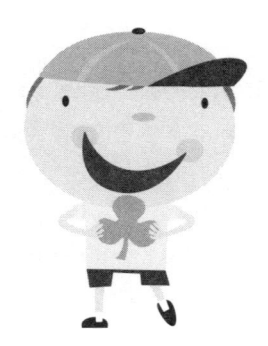

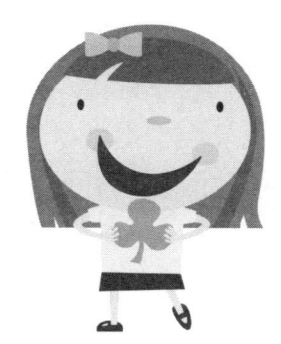

More recently, the International Study of Asthma and Allergic Conditions (ISAAC) studies, a series of large, population-based investigations using validated questionnaires designed to compare asthma prevalence between countries and to assess changes in epidemiology over time. Initially, children aged thirteen to fourteen years were studied, but younger groups, aged six to seven years, were subsequently included. The initial Irish study showed that asthma prevalence in thirteen-to fourteen-year-olds was 15.2 percent in 1995 and by 2007 had risen to 21.6 percent, a relative increase of 33 percent. Ireland comes fourth in an international league table of asthma prevalence, behind Australia, New Zealand and the UK. Follow-up ISAAC studies have generally shown no significant increases in many areas, with existing high prevalence giving rise to some authorities suggesting that the prevalence is plateauing in these regions. However, increases have been observed in regions that had low prevalence rates in the initial assessment.

In Ireland, the burden of asthma is high, with one in five Irish schoolchildren having asthma symptoms. The condition affects one-eighth of the general population, and it is estimated that there are 470,000 asthma sufferers in Ireland. There are 5,500 admissions every year; 55 percent are less than fourteen years old. There are approximately eighty adult deaths per year due to asthma. Thirty percent of these were less than forty years of age. Fortunately, deaths in children from asthma are relatively rare, usually less than one per year.

In a study published in 2005, four hundred patients with current asthma in Ireland were interviewed in the Asthma Insights and Reality in Ireland (AIRI) survey to determine their health-care utilisation, symptom severity, activity limitations and level of asthma control. Of those surveyed, acute services were utilised by a significant number of respondents. Over the previous year, 27 percent had either an emergency visit to the hospital or their general practitioner (GP), and 7 percent were hospitalised for asthma. In terms of asthma control, 19 percent experienced sleep disturbance at least once a week, 29 percent missed work or school, and 37 percent of respondents experienced symptoms during physical activity over the previous four-week period. Based on these findings, the level of asthma control and asthma management in Ireland falls well short of recommended national and international asthma guidelines.

In a similar study in 2010, the market research company Rollercoaster conducted a survey of 271 randomly ascertained children with asthma. It was found that 92 percent of parents were satisfied or very satisfied with their child's asthma control. Dispite this, 35 percent used their rescue inhaler either daily or weekly. Furthermore 59 percent experienced night-time awakenings, 25 percent have exercise limited days and 26 percent miss school on either daily or weekly basis. There still appears to be a disconnect between parental perception of asthma symptoms and actual control using accepted clinical criteria. This is a worrying trend

The economic burden of asthma in Ireland is substantial. In 2003, the total cost to the state was €463 million, and emergency care and hospitalisation accounted for €227 million (49 percent) of this. In adults, almost twelve working days a year are lost to asthma. This figure does not include the parents who miss work to care for children with asthma. In 2009, it was estimated that one million school days were lost due to asthma. A survey of the published data on the costs of childhood asthma conducted in 2004 showed that costs vary widely across the European Union. The study found that the direct and indirect costs of childhood asthma in Ireland amount to an average of €613 per child each year. This compares to €269 in the UK, €300 in France, €429 in Finland and €559 in Holland.

What causes asthma?

The simple answer is that we don't know what causes asthma. If you would like to get an overview of recent theories on asthma, please read on. From the 1930s to the 1950s, asthma was considered as being one of the 'holy seven' psychosomatic illnesses. Its cause was considered to be psychological, with treatment often based on psychoanalysis. As these psychoanalysts interpreted the asthmatic wheeze as the suppressed cry of the child for its mother, so they considered that the treatment of depression was especially important for individuals with asthma.

Many hypotheses have been proposed relating to the causes of asthma, but it is unlikely that there is a single explanation. It is probable that asthma develops as the result of a complex interaction between genes responsible for allergy and bronchial hyper-responsiveness and the environment. One of the difficulties with genetic and epidemiological studies is disease definition. It is likely that there is not a single form of asthma. The clinical expression of any genetic abnormality is known as a phenotype. Increasingly it is being recognised that there are probably many variations of asthma phenotypes, symptom clusters and other associated atopic conditions. This is also true for trigger factors, and responses to treatment: e.g. asthma, eczema and rhinitis combination, aspirin-sensitive asthma and nasal polyps, isolated exercise-induced asthma, pre-school virus-triggered wheeze and non-allergic asthma in adults.

Autonomic imbalance

The autonomic nervous system (ANS) is the part of the nervous system that controls bodily functions in an unconscious fashion. It continues to function during sleep and coma. The ANS affects heart rate, digestion, respiration rate, salivation, perspiration, pupil reactions, urination and sexual arousal. Whereas most of its actions are involuntary, some such as breathing work in tandem with the conscious mind.

The ANS is classically divided into two subsystems: the parasympathetic and sympathetic nervous system. Relatively recently, a third subsystem of neurons (called 'non-adrenergic and non-cholinergic' neurons) have been described; these have been found to be integral in autonomic function, particularly in the gut and the lungs. Before we understood the inflammatory nature of asthma, it was hypothesised by some that asthma was caused by an imbalance between the sympathetic (bronchodilator) and parasympathetic (brochoconstrictor) systems. The normal calibre of the bronchus is maintained by complex reflex interactions between the systems. The parasympathetic reflex loop consists of nerve endings, which originate under the inner lining of the bronchus. Whenever these nerve endings are stimulated via the inflamed mucosa (for example, by dust, cold air or fumes), sensory impulses travel via the vagus nerve to the brainstem, then down the vagal motor pathway, to reach the bronchial small airways again. Acetylcholine is released from the efferent nerve endings. This acetylcholine results in the excessive formation of inositol 1,4,5-trisphosphate (IP3) in bronchial smooth muscle cells, which leads to muscle shortening. Thus, excess parasympathetic stimulation initiates broncho-constriction.

On the other hand, the sympathetic nervous system is regulated by chemicals like adrenalin, nor-adrenalin and isoprenalin, which cause a widening of the airway by relaxing bronchial smooth muscle. Interestingly, in the 1960s in former USSR, vagotomy was employed to remove excessive parasympathetic input as a means of treating asthma. Nowadays, most of the drugs used to relieve acute asthma symptoms either stimulate the sympathetic nervous system (e.g. Salbutamol) or antagonise the parasympathetic nervous system (e.g. Ipratroprium).]

Genetics

The familial tendency to asthma was recognised as early as the eleventh century. In the late 1980s, as advances in genetic science were made, an inheritance pattern for atopy was proposed. If neither parent was affected, the chance of the offspring being allergic was 14 percent. If one parent was affected, the risk rose to 50 percent, and if both parents were affected, the chances increased to almost 80 percent. Not all studies have confirmed these risks, and the disparity may be explained by a genetic phenomenon called imprinting, whereby the risk is stronger when a mother is affected. However, the maternal influence on the development of atopy could also be explained by foetal allergen exposures in the womb. In general, studies in identical twins are often used to determine the strength of a genetic component on the risk of disease development. If genetic influences are strong, there will be a high level of concordance of a given condition in the twins. In large studies of newborn identical twins, the levels of IgE are consistent; however, the rates of asthma within the twin pairs differ considerably, suggesting that environmental factors must be important.

Certain unique populations have been identified where rates of asthma are very high. One such population lives on the remote South Atlantic island of Tristan da Cunha, where asthma and bronchial hyper-responsiveness are highly prevalent. This isolated, genetically homogenous (in-bred) population is descended from two original settlers, who were mutineers from the infamous British naval ship *The Bounty*. Asthma-prevalence rates on the island were almost 60 percent. Asthma is also very common amongst New Zealand Maoris, who appear to have a more severe form of the condition. A number of studies in asymptomatic infants have shown high levels of bronchial hyper-responsiveness, which tends to diminish with age. Why it persists in some is unclear, but it is probably related to their atopic tendency and early environmental exposures. A number of investigators have linked candidate genes to bronchial hyper-responsiveness, and some of these genes are located in close proximity to a cluster on chromosome 5 linked to the presence of atopy. There is a group of proteins now known as the ADAM superfamily. ADAM 33, a member of this family of genes, encodes a subgroup of zinc dependent proteinases, which may be important in asthma. Mutations in this gene have been associated with the tendency to bronchial hyper-responsiveness. The potential for therapeutic intervention with ADAM 33 is extremely attractive, and further work will focus not only on the specific domains of ADAM 33 but also the mechanisms by which they lead to bronchial hyper-reactivity. However, this gene is only one of forty-three thus far associated with asthma. Others include genes that code for cytokines involved in the inflammatory or allergic process e.g. tumour necrosis factor alpha, interleukin-4, or toll-like receptors, whilst others are involved in the sympathetic nervous response e.g. receptor subunits. There are likely to be important modifier genes, which modulate the ultimate expression of phenotype.

In 2010 a study published in the New England Journal of Medicine reported the results of the Consortium-based genomewide association study of asthma. They evaluated 10,000 asthmatics and 16,000 individuals without asthma. They looked at almost 600,000 subtle genetic mutations (single nucleotide polymorphisms) in each person. They identified nine important loci (genetic regions), which were previously not associated with asthma. One particular region was associated with childhood-onset asthma. Interestingly, there were no particularly strong links with loci involved with IgE production leading commentators to suggest that atopy/allergy is probably only an association with asthma, not the underlying cause.

Genetics may also explain how we differ in our response to asthma medications (agonists, antileukotrienes and corticosteroids). Already we know that some of us carry mutations in the gene that codes part of the receptor for drugs like Salbutamol, which means that in some cases we may react to it in a suboptimum way, or have a paradoxical response.

Early-exposure theories

Most asthma presents before six years of age. It is now believed that our immune system goes through a window period in early life (possibly in the womb) where exposure to infections, irritants or allergens may dictate the outcome later in childhood. In fact, maternal pre-conceptual allergen avoidance has been studied, in the hope that it may lead to fewer babies born with allergies and asthma. Most clinical trials that have looked at this question to date have been disappointing in that they have failed to show any significant beneficial effect.

The role of breastfeeding in asthma prevention is probably beneficial. Breast feeding is superior to bottle feeding and is recommended for many other reasons, including improved nutrition, less gastro-intestinal infection, better maternal-infant bonding, and higher neuro-cognative outcomes. Breastfed babies get fewer chest infections while being breastfed, but this effect wears off once breastfeeding has been stopped. This protective effect is extremely beneficial in under-developed countries, where infant mortality rates are very high, and respiratory infection is a leading cause of death. In developed counties, data from the Tucson Birth Cohort suggests that breastfeeding for four to six months protects against the development of asthma and allergies in most cases. However, there was a small group of infants born to atopic mothers where breastfeeding increased the risk. Some suggest that the mechanism for this phenomenon is the transmission of IgE (maternally-derived, biologically active milk) in breast milk, which is allergy-producing in the infant. Thus we have a situation where an atopic mother breastfeeds with the intention of preventing allergies/asthma but unintentionally increases the infant's chances of developing these conditions. Introduction of solid foods at four to six months is not associated with increased allergy/asthma in the general population.

It has been known that maternal smoking during pregnancy causes low birth-weight babies. It is not as widely recognised that this exposure results in babies with narrow-calibre airways that are more prone to wheeze. Babies born to smoking mothers have higher IgE levels. Maternal paracetamol consumption during pregnancy has been also linked to asthma and elevated IgE risk in later childhood. High levels of dust mite from carpets and soft furnishing in the home during infancy have been shown to be strongly associated with the risk of asthma in later childhood. Infections with respiratory syncytial virus, which causes bronchiolitis (a wheezing illness in babies), has been shown to be associated with asthma in later childhood. Some authorities suggest that this virus is asthmagenic, whereas most people believe that RSV only produces bronchiolitis in those infants with weaker lungs. In other words, babies get bronchiolitis because they are prone to asthma in the first place.

The hygiene hypothesis was first proposed by Dr David Strachan, a UK epidemiologist, in an article published in the *British Medical Journal*, in 1989. The hygiene hypothesis was proposed to explain the observation that allergic diseases were less common in children from larger families, which were presumably exposed to more infectious agents through their siblings, than in children from families with only one child. The hygiene hypothesis has been extensively investigated by researchers and has become an important paradigm for the study of allergic disorders. It forms the basis for the observed increase in allergic diseases following industrialisation, and a higher incidence of allergic diseases in more developed countries. The hygiene hypothesis has now been expanded to include exposure to micro-organisms such as symbiotic bacteria and parasites as important modulators of immunity. The hypothesis also suggests that, in the absence of infestations and significant early infection, a switch occurs in our immune system that enables the excess production of the allergy antibody IgE rather than our normal protective antibody, IgG.

The science behind this theory suggests that, in the absence of the appropriate immunological stimuli early in life, a critical switch occurs with failure to develop mature T-regulatory lymphocytes, thus allowing excess proliferation of Th2 lymphocytes, which synthesize cytokines, promoting excess IgE production and the proliferation of mast cells and eosinophils that are key effectors of allergic inflammation. IgE is a critical driver of allergic inflammation. As a result of this hypothesis, interest has developed in helminthic therapy, a type of immunotherapy involving parasitic worms such as hookworms and whipworms. It has been proposed that helminthic therapy can successfully treat allergic and autoimmune disorders via deliberate infestation with a wild-type helminth or with their ova or cells components, which are known to be allergenic.

Socio-economic conditions play a role in asthma and allergies, and for many years allergies were considered afflictions of the affluent. In fact, researchers have shown that there are close correlations between a country's GDP and the prevalence of allergies and asthma. In underdeveloped countries, where asthma prevalence is generally low, and rates of natural infection are high, the antibody IgE is primarily concerned with the containment of parasites within the gut and the prevention of their dissemination throughout the body. The theory goes that in developed countries, where infection rates are low and parasitic infestation extremely rare, the IgE system has become unnecessary, and thus atopy diseases are the by-products of this redundancy. There have been several epidemiological studies from the UK, Italy, Israel and the US, which looked at asthma prevalence in immigrants from underdeveloped countries with low rates of asthma. The data generally shows that second-generation immigrants born in a developed country are more likely to describe regular asthma symptoms and be on regular inhaler treatment, but that for those born abroad; there is an increasing rate of symptoms and medication use, with increasing duration of residence in the country.

Data from epidemiological studies support this theory: younger children from big families have fewer allergies; the number of viral infections in early life is protective against the development of asthma; and infants who attend crèche are at lower risk than those cared for at home. In contrast to what was previously thought, children who are exposed in early life to pets or farmyard animals have a reduced risk of asthma/allergy. Higher levels of endotoxin (derived from bacterial cell walls) found in house dust was associated with lower rates of allergic response. There appears to be an urban/rural divide, in that rates of asthma and allergy tend to be higher in those who live in cities. Growing up on a farm also appears to be protective. Although not recommended, the regular consumption of non-pasteurised milk, and failure to receive childhood vaccinations, are statistically associated with lower levels of allergy and asthma. Our affluent Western lifestyle means that we are healthier and our children no longer die in large numbers from infectious diseases. However, there may be a price that our population has to pay for this. The strongest evidence in support of the hygiene hypothesis comes from studies comparing asthma and allergy prevalence in the former East Germany and West Germany. They found lower rates of asthma/allergy in East Germany, where infection rates and industrial air pollution were high. At follow-up, ten years after unification, socio-economic conditions had improved in the former East Germany, and rates of asthma/allergy had increased and were equivalent to those in the former West Germany.

Vitamin D theory
An intriguing hypothesis on asthma/allergies has been proposed recently, which suggests that Vitamin D deficiency, or insufficiency, may play an important role in the development of asthma. It is now recognised that Vitamin D is not merely a vitamin. It chemically resembles the naturally occurring steroid hormones, synthetic forms of which are used in the treatment of inflammation. Vitamin D is ingested in food but is also produced in the skin on exposure to sunlight. It is now widely accepted that it is a potent immunomodulator and has been shown to dampen inflammation in laboratory experiments. Vitamin D intake in pregnancy appears to have an influence on the infant's tendency to respiratory infection and subsequent wheeze later in childhood.

Some investigators have shown links between maternal Vitamin D and asthma. In third world countries Vitamin D deficiency is associated with higher rates of respiratory illness. Our own work has shown that Vitamin D plays an important role in the modulation of airway inflammation on children with cystic fibrosis. It stimulates the release of cathelicidin, which is a natural antimicrobial peptide that helps the body overcome bacterial infections. In a recent study from Japan, Vitamin D supplementation protected against epidemic forms of influenza A.

Urban children are less active, prone to obesity, and spend more time indoors watching TV and playing video games. They consume a calorie-rich diet that is relatively low in Vitamin D. The hypothesis proposes that these factors combine to produce Vitamin D insufficiency, which in turn predisposes them to asthma. Critics argue that bad asthma can lead to inactivity etc., and that Vitamin D is merely a reflection, not the cause of bad asthma, and that this is what is termed 'an epi-phenomenon'

However, many epidemiological studies in children and adults with asthma have shown a strong link between asthma severity, degree of allergy, and Vitamin D insufficiency. A recently published study in Polish children demonstrated some interesting trends; those children who received Vitamin D supplements at a dose of 500iu daily, as well as an inhaled steroid, appeared to have better outcomes in terms of asthma control, compared to children who received the inhaled steroid, alone. However, this study size was small and the dose of Vitamin D quite low. Although further studies are underway, at the time of writing routine supplementation with Vitamin D is not recommended for improving asthma control.

Chlorinated swimming pools

Field sports, particularly during the cold winter months, can often trigger asthma symptoms. This is thought to be due to the effects of fast breathing and cold, damp or very dry air. For many years, swimming was recommended as an exercise for people with asthma. The rationale was that the air was warm and humid in an indoor pool, and thus was less irritating to the lungs. Many people found that they could exercise quite vigorously without developing any asthma symptoms. However, recent research has suggested that repeated exposure to chlorine in pools may induce asthma in children.

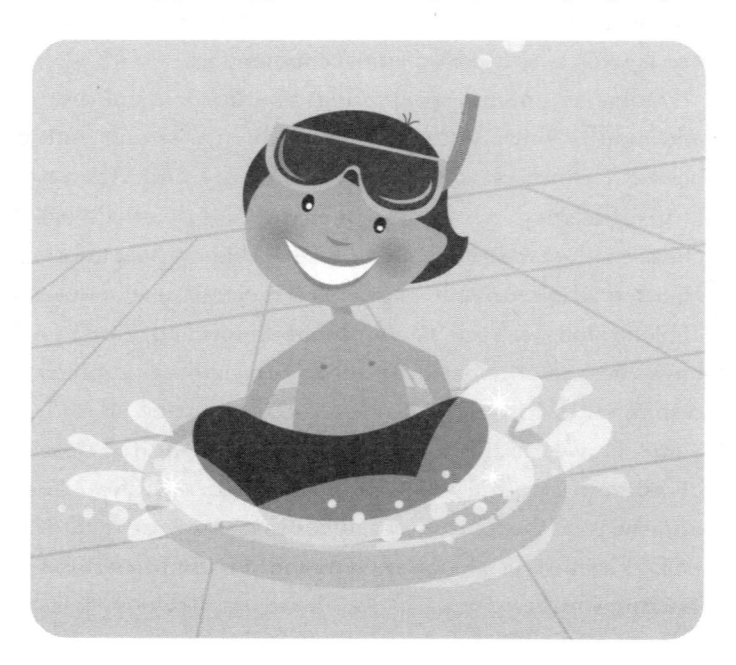

It has been known for some time that acute accidental exposure to high levels of chlorine gas causes asthma symptoms. Repeated exposure to lower levels of chlorine in elite swimmers, pool attendants and swim coaches has also been reported to cause asthma. The chlorinated swimming pool hypothesis, first proposed by a group of medical researchers led by Professor Alfred Bernard of the University of Louvain in Belgium in 2003, was that asthma may be induced in the young by repeated exposure to chlorine-related compounds from swimming pools. The hypothesis was supported by an epidemiological study based in a cohort of pre-school children and their exposure to swimming pools. It is also known that chlorine reacts with human proteins in pool water to produce the vapour trichloramine, which lies just above the water. Laboratory experiments have shown that trichloramine can produce harmful effects on the integrity of the lining of the bronchial tubes, disruption of the mucosa or lining of the airway, which normally acts as protective barrier against various germs, and may permit airborne allergens to cross this barrier.

In his study of 341 schoolchildren, Bernard found that long-term attendance at indoor chlorinated swimming pools up to the age of about six to seven years was a strong predictor of airway inflammation, while for those children who were atopic, the total time spent at indoor chlorinated swimming pools was a strong predictor of the risk of developing asthma. In a later study of 190,000 children in twenty-one countries in Europe, conducted by the same group, it was found that thirteen- to fourteen-year-old children were 2 to 3.5 percent more likely to have or have had asthma for every additional indoor chlorinated pool per 100,000 inhabitants in their place of residence. These investigations have provoked significant debate within the scientific community.

However in 2010, a prospective longitudinal study was conducted that followed 5,738 British children. Data on swimming was collected by questionnaire at 6, 18, 38, 42, 57, 65 and 81 months, in order to examine whether swimming in infancy and childhood was associated with asthma and allergic symptoms at age seven and ten years. Information on rhinitis, wheezing, asthma, eczema, hay fever, and asthma medications was collected by questionnaire at seven and ten years. Lung function and allergy testing were performed at seven years. They found that at age seven, over 50 percent of the children swam at least once per week. Swimming frequency did not increase the risk of symptoms, either overall or in allergic children. Children with a high versus low cumulative swimming pool attendance from birth to seven years had similar risks for the current asthma or 'asthma ever' at age seven years. Similar findings were observed at age ten years. They concluded that chlorinated pool swimming did not increase the risk of asthma or allergic symptoms in British children and that swimming was associated with increased lung function and lower risk of asthma symptoms, especially among children with pre-existing respiratory conditions.

Air pollution

Air pollution in developed countries is mainly caused by exhausts from cars and factories, smoke and road dust. When inhaled, outdoor pollutants can aggravate the lungs, and can lead to chest pain, coughing, shortness of breath and throat irritation. On days when air pollution is highest, there are increased hospital admissions, with patients suffering from all forms of respiratory disorders. In an elegant study, asthmatic subjects were asked to walk for two hours in Hyde Park or Oxford Street in London. Those assigned Oxford Street experienced a drop in their pulmonary function tests and increased markers of airway inflammation compared to the other group. It is now widely accepted that air pollution worsens chronic respiratory diseases, such as asthma and chronic obstructive pulmonary disease. However, there is still considerable debate as to whether air pollution can actually cause asthma.

Particulate matter, carbon monoxide and nitrogen dioxide are often used as a measure of the intensity of vehicle emissions. In two separate studies published in 2008, German and Swedish epidemiologists found a significant relationship between allergic sensitisation and wheeze with early and prolonged exposure to high levels of particulate matter and nitrogen dioxide. High levels of traffic emissions in Copenhagen were associated with an increased risk of wheeze within the first three years of life of a birth cohort. Several studies have demonstrated a higher prevalence of asthma in children and adults who reside in close proximity to major roads and motorways. In experiments, mice exposed to diesel exhausts developed abnormalities of their immune system, which led to an allergy response and increased IgE production. If applicable to humans, this mechanism may explain the emerging relationship between traffic pollution and higher levels of asthma.

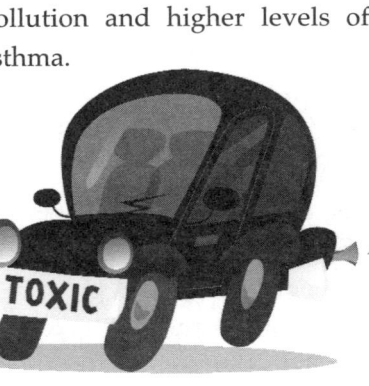

Obesity

The increase in asthma prevalence has occurred with a parallel increase in the rate of occurrence of obesity in developed countries. Many studies have linked the two conditions both in children and in adults. Fat or adipose tissue is no longer considered an inert body component. It is now known that fat cells release hormone-like substances and inflammatory mediators that may have an important effect on metabolism. Thus, it is suggested that the obese state itself may cause or contribute to the development of asthma. Several studies have shown that obesity predisposes to the development of asthma particularly in adolescent females. Data from the Tucson Birth Cohort indicates that females who become obese before adolescence have a high risk of developing asthma.

In our own study performed in healthy prepubertal Irish school children, 25 percent were found to be overweight/obese. A notable minority of children already had significant risk factors for cardiac disease in adulthood such as high cholesterol and elevated blood pressure. We also found that pre-adolescent females take significantly less exercise and are more overweight than their male peers.

The mechanism for the association between obesity and asthma is unclear. Obesity can restrict lung capacity, reduce the calibre of peripheral airways and potentially increase bronchial hyper-responsiveness. Markers of inflammation are higher in obese subjects and some investigators have shown important correlations between them and the degree of asthma severity. Obese patients with asthma may respond less well to corticosteroid treatment. They have lower Vitamin D levels than those of normal weight. It is very likely that more than one biological explanation underlies the association between the two. Weight management is advocated as an important component of care for asthmatic children.

Gastro-oesophageal reflux (GOR)

Gastro-oesophageal reflux is a condition where the contents of the stomach and gastric acid move back up into the gullet because of weakness of the sphincter muscle that acts as a valve between the two. GOR in adults presents as indigestion and heartburn. It is often treated with antacids available over the counter. In children, and those with asthma, it can often be asymptomatic and only detected by a test called twenty-four-hour lower oesophageal pH monitoring. The relationship between the two is unclear. Some authorities suggest that a causal relationship exists between asthma and GOR. In animal models, increased airway resistance results in a greater transpulmonary pressure (negative pressure within the thorax) leading to deficient function of the lower oesophageal sphincter and GOR. Acid reflux on inflamed oesophageal mucosa can induce broncho-constriction. Aspiration of refluxed gastric contents can contribute to airway inflammation and provoke an acute episode. Despite this evidence, there has not been a satisfactory clinical trial showing that treatment of asymptomatic GOR alters the outcome in terms of asthma control.

What are the common triggers?

Each person differs in terms of their specific triggers. It is important for each patient (or their parent) to identify their own trigger factors and take the necessary avoidance measures where possible. Optimum control of the bronchial inflammation reduces a child's susceptibility to a given trigger.

Viral upper respiratory tract infections are the most common trigger. In normal children they result in just snuffles and colds, or tickly coughs that last only a couple of days and settle without treatment. In a child with poorly controlled asthma a trivial head cold can result in a severe attack. Exercise can trigger cough, wheeze, chest tightness or breathlessness in otherwise well controlled people with asthma. More commonly exercise-induced symptoms reflect poorly controlled asthma i.e. there will be symptoms unrelated to exertion, and this indicates that there is a need to increase an individuals controller therapy. More rarely, isolated activity-induced asthma is observed, which requires a different management approach (see exercise-induced asthma).

Fumes from gas or coal fires, sprays from aerosols, paint fumes, Christmas trees, or tobacco smoke can all set off an episode of asthma. Exposure to allergens such as house dust mite, grass pollen, animal hair (dog, cat and horse) and moulds can trigger asthma and allergic rhinitis. Moulds arise from damp housing conditions with obvious mildew or during house renovations where fungal spores are released from old plasterwork. Both are known to contribute to increased respiratory illness and asthma symptoms. A common scenario is where a dust allergic child develops an asthma attack having spent a night in either a holiday home/caravan, a grandparent's house or on a sleep-over at a friend's house. Conditions at these locations may be dusty and thus trigger an asthma attack.

Ingested substances such as aspirin, NSAIDs (like neurofen), carbonated drinks, tatrazine, sulphites, aspartame, metabisulphite, monosodium glutamate and food colourants have all been documented as triggers for asthma episodes. Cold drinks or ice cream may trigger an episode via stimulation of the vagus nerve through receptors in the oesophagus. Bronchospasm can occur as part of a generalised reaction to food in anaphylaxis, e.g. a peanut allergy.

> **How is asthma diagnosed?**

Asthma is usually diagnosed using clinical skills (patient history and examination) by your GP. Initially a history will be taken. Recurrent symptoms such as dry cough, wheeze or breathlessness are suggestive of the diagnosis (see question 10 for more details). A personal history of eczema or allergic rhinitis would also be supportive. A child's height and weight are measured and then plotted on a centile chart. These would be expected to be normal. The respiratory examination may be entirely normal. The hands are checked for finger clubbing, which is observed in some chronic respiratory disorders but never in asthma. Sometimes if the condition has persisted for a long time, changes will occur in the shape of the chest. A pigeon-shaped breastbone (Pectus carinatum) with indrawing of the lower ribs (Harrison's sulci) may be observed in some patients. Sometimes children with asthma have a hollow breastbone (pectus excavatum). There may be pallor, swelling and mucous coating of the lining of the nasal passages suggesting allergic rhinitis. Nasal polyps are quite rare in children with nasal allergy. The may be a transverse nasal crease due to constant rubbing of the nose. Frequently, examination with the stethoscope will be normal. However, during an asthma episode wheeze can be heard and the breath sounds may be decreased in more severe attacks. A bluish discoloration of the lips and tongue (cyanosis) may be apparent when oxygen levels in the bloodstream are low.

A peak-flow measurement can be taken in older more co-operative children. The reading may be lower than expected for the child's height, sex and age. If so, bronchodilators like Ventolin® can be given to see if it improves. Sometimes your GP may give a therapeutic trial of asthma treatment in a younger child that is suspected to have asthma. Unfortunately there is no such thing as an asthma test. There are a number of additional tests that one can undergo to confirm a clinical suspicion of asthma. A Chest X-ray is frequently normal or may show slight thickening of the bronchial tubes and increased inflation of the lungs. A chest X-ray is not used to diagnose asthma but may, in some circumstances, help exclude conditions which may mimic asthma. Sometimes your GP may consider making a referral to a respiratory or allergy specialist, who in turn may order allergy or pulmonary function tests to facilitate the diagnostic process.

How is asthma control assessed?

Your doctor will frequently use research-based treatment guidelines to assess and treat your child's asthma. These guidelines are updated regularly to keep up with advances in medicine. Asthma control is usually assessed using a composite of the patient history, examination, validated questionnaire, peak flow rate and pulmonary function tests. A useful self-administered test is the childhood asthma control test (see www.asthmacontrol.com/child.html), which assess asthma control over the previous four weeks in aged either four to twelve years or older than twelve years.

The absence of symptoms, infrequent use of rescue medication (bronchodilator), normal exercise tolerance, normal pulmonary function and few missed school days are generally signs that the asthma is well controlled. Infrequent or lack of exacerbations (asthma attacks) also suggests that asthma is under control. If asthma is under good control your doctor may attempt to reduce (step down) your child's controller medications. If control has been good for long periods, pulmonary function tests are normal and your child is on minimal doses of preventative treatment it may be decided to give your child a trial off therapy.

Asthma that is not controlled is characterised by frequent symptoms and use of rescue medication, more frequent asthma attacks, courses of oral steroids and antibiotics, poor school attendance and abnormal pulmonary function. When asthma is poorly controlled the patient needs to be re-evaluated. It must be ascertained that they are avoiding their specific triggers e.g. second-hand tobacco smoke, that they are taking their controller medication regularly, using the correct device for the age and developmental status, and using their device correctly. If the clinician is satisfied that the child is receiving the medication correctly, then a step-up in dose will be made or other treatments may be added in. Once control has been achieved for at least three months, then a step down may be considered.

What are asthma guidelines?

Many guidelines have been made available to help clinicians manage asthma in a systematic way e.g. GINA, BTS/SIGN and PractALL. In these islands, the most commonly referred to guidelines in this part of the World are the GINA and BTS/SIGN guidelines.

The Global Initiative for Asthma (GINA) works with health care professionals and public health officials around the world to reduce asthma prevalence, morbidity, and mortality. GINA was launched in 1993 in collaboration with the National Heart, Lung, and Blood Institute; National Institutes of Health, USA; and the World Health Organisation. GINA aims to improve the lives of people with asthma throughout the world. In order to have more uniform management of asthma on a global scale, GINA has developed guidelines for treatment of adult and children's asthma based on the best available research. These step-based guidelines can facilitate doctors caring for asthma patients. The evidence-based guidelines are updated regularly, information on which can be found at www.ginasthma.com. GINA promotes events such World Asthma Day, which is usually held on the first Tuesday in May. The British Thoracic Society and the Scottish Intercollegiate Guideline Network produce similar treatment guidelines, which are available at www.sign.ac.uk

Both guidelines are quite similar in terms of their aims. Although there are subtle differences in emphasis, the treatment recommendations they do not differ greatly. The aim of asthma management is control of the disease. In both sets of guidelines asthma is treated according to the age of the child (separate for those under five years, and aged five to twelve years). Both guidelines stress the importance of trigger avoidance, adherence to prescribed treatment and appropriateness of the inhalation device with the correct technique.

Asthma is then characterised as being controlled or not. If asthma has been controlled for the previous three to six months, it may be possible to reduce the amount of medication taken. This is known as stepping down. If the opposite situation applies then it may be necessary to increase medication, which is known as stepping up. Asthma is recognised as being a variable condition and thus an individual patient may go through periods of good or poor control where their medication is stepped up or down where appropriate.

Examples of the guidelines are as follows: in children over five years old, Step 1 is where asthma is infrequent, mild and episodic. This level of asthma is treated with an inhaled short-acting bronchodilator like Ventolin® as required. The next level is Step 2, where symptoms are more persistent and bronchodilator is being used more than twice per week. An inhaled steroid is added at low-dose e.g. Beclomethasone 100 or equivalent twice daily. The next level is Step 3, where there are three choices: firstly, to double the dose of inhaled steroid. Secondly add a long acting bronchodilator, or thirdly, add an antileukotriene drug. Step 4 involves using higher dose of inhaled steroids. Step 5 involves using regular oral steroids and possibly trying drugs like Xolair® (Anti-IgE). The major difference between the guidelines is at Step 3: those over five years where the BTS/Sign guidelines have a preference of the additional of LABA, whereas the GINA guideline also includes the antileukotriene and low dose slow release theophylline option. In those under five years, both guidelines recommend a six-to-eight-week trial of antileukotriene at Step 2 as an alternative to starting an inhaled corticosteroid and as a controller where activity-induced symptoms are a particularly problematic.

Summary of stepwise management in children aged five to twelve years

Step 1: Mild intermittent asthma

* As required short acting bronchodilator

Step 2: Mild persistent asthma

* As in Step 1, plus the addition of an inhaled steroid 200 to 400 mcg/day*

* (Other preventer drug if inhaled steroid cannot be used, e.g. LTRA or cromolyn)

*If control is still inadequate, institute trial of other therapies, such as leukotriene receptor antagonist or SR theophylline

- ✳ 200 mcg is an appropriate starting dose for many patients
- ✳ Start at dose of inhaled steroid appropriate to severity of disease.

Step 3: Moderate persistent asthma

- ✳ As in Step 2, plus the addition of inhaled long-acting-beta-agonist (LABA)
- **A** reassess control of asthma: if good response to LABA - continue LABA
- **B** benefit from LABA but control still inadequate
- **C** continue LABA and increase inhaled steroid dose to 400 mcg/day* (if not already on this dose)
- **D** no response to LABA - stop LABA and increase inhaled steroid to 400 mcg/ day.

*If control is still inadequate, institute trial of other therapies, such as leukotriene receptor antagonist or SR theophylline

Step 4: Severe persistent asthma

- ✳ Initial add-on therapy: Increase inhaled steroid up to 800 mcg/day*

Step 5: Persistent poor control

- ✳ Use daily steroid tablet in lowest dose providing adequate control
- ✳ Maintain high dose inhaled steroid at 800 mcg/day*

Consider referral to respiratory paediatrician at Step 3 or beyond.

*Beclomethasone or equivalent

> **Which device is right?**

For asthma to be adequately controlled it is vital that the correct device is prescribed and that parents and the child understand the correct way to use it. Generally speaking, the most effective asthma treatments are best delivered by the inhaled route where the drug gets to the lung directly as opposed to oral treatments. Tablets or liquids have to be swallowed and progress into the stomach, then absorbed into the bloodstream and passed to the lung and other tissues. The doses of oral treatment tend to be higher and there is a greater potential for side effects.

The device your child will be prescribed will depend on their age and developmental progress. For uncooperative infants and toddlers, spacing devices with a face-mask (Aerochamber®, Babyhaler®) are the first choice. These devices deliver some drug to the lung but a large proportion of each inhalation (98-99 percent) remains either in the chamber, mouth or is swallowed. If using inhaled steroids it is better to use one of the more modern agents that have low systemic bioavailability (are not active once swallowed). Studies have shown that a child who struggles with the mask or who screams throughout administration will not receive an effective dose of medication. Some infants will tolerate a spacer and mask only while asleep. Some toddlers will tolerate an initial dose via the spacer, but later start to resist. In this case your doctor may want to use a higher concentration inhaler in order to give the same dose to your child with fewer puffs.

It is important to rinse the mouth with a drink and wipe the face with a damp cloth following the administration of an inhaled steroid in order to reduce the risk of facial rash and oral thrush. Large volume spacers (Volumatic®, Nebuhaler®) are suitable for children aged three and a half years and older. Although bulkier, they have the advantage of delivering more of the drug to the lower airways than infant spacers. These spacers need to be maintained carefully; each week they should be soaked in soapy water, rinsed and drained. Wiping spacers dry with dish cloth is not recommended because this can increase the static charge on the inside of the device, more of the inhaled drug sticks to the inner surface, which in turn interferes with amount of the medication delivered to the airways. That is why it is recommended that the new or recently cleaned spacers be primed with several puffs of inhaler before the drug is actually administered to the child. Once children reach school age, dry powder devices (Turbohaler®, Accuhaler®) become an option. They are smaller, more portable and deliver equivalent amounts of drug to the lower airways. Excellent video-streams which demonstrate the correct inhaler technique for the various devices are available on the Asthma Society's of Ireland website www.asthmasociety.ie

Tips for giving a young child their inhaler

If the infant or toddler refuses the mask then one can try to give it during sleep. Nebulisers are sometimes used in this age group, however they take longer to administer medications (five to ten minutes), frequently require an A/C power supply and generate a lot of noise, which means that they can be less acceptable in some children of this age. Sometimes when inhalation therapy is not feasible because of poor co-operation, a trial of oral treatment may be recommended.

How to use a Babyhaler or Aerochamber (with mask)

Shake the metered dose inhaler before use. Attach it to the chamber. Place the mask over the nose and mouth. Ensure that there is a tight seal. Keep the device level. Press on the inhaler ONCE. Keep the mask in position for ten seconds (count one-one thousand, two-one thousand, etc). A break can be taken if your baby needs one. Repeat the procedure if further puffs are required. Wipe your child's face with a damp cloth and give them a drink after that inhaler session.

Remember: 'A good start is half the battle'. Let your child become familiar with the spacer and inhaler. Let them play with the spacer and if necessary allow them chew and dribble on it. The devices are quite hardy and can always be washed. Allow your child play with the inhaler even waste a few sprays so that they'll know what to expect when you are actually going to give the medication. Never try to give the inhaler when your child is tired, irritable, hungry, or wants to do something else. Be patient and do not force the device over the child's face. Sometimes putting colourful stickers on the device make it less frightening for the child. It can be a good idea to watch a favourite video, read a picture book or sing a nursery rhyme when actually giving the inhalers. It may be necessary to take a break between inhalations. Reward co-operation.

How to use a Volumatic, Nebuhaler or Aerochamber (with mouthpiece)

Assemble the two halves of the device. Shake the metered dose inhaler before use. Fit the inhaler into the aperture. Place your lips around the mouth piece. Depress the inhaler once. Your child should take 5 slow breaths for each puff required. It is important to exhale before taking the next breath in. Panting into the device is not effective. Watch the devices valve open and close. Repeat the procedure if further puffs are required. Once the inhaler session is complete, rinse your mouth or brush your teeth or have a drink to remove any drug from the mouth.

How to use dry-powder inhalers (Diskus® or Turbohaler®)

Diskus: open the device. Slide the lever away from you until you hear a click. Exhale fully before placing your mouth around the mouthpiece. Inhale deeply and hold your breath for approximately ten seconds, then exhale. Do not exhale into the device. The Diskus has a dose counter that indicates how many doses remain. Close the device. Repeat the procedure if further doses are required

Turbohaler: Unscrew and remove the white cover. Load by holding the inhaler upright. Twist the grip fully in one direction and back again until you hear a click. Exhale deeply and then place your mouth over the mouth piece. Inhale deeply and hold your breath for approximately ten seconds, then exhale. Do not exhale into the device.

> **'Majority Of Patients May Be Using Prescribed Medication Inhalers Incorrectly!'**
> REUTERS (Feb 10th 2011)

Reuters recently reported a study by Norton and colleagues who found that many people with diseases such as emphysema or asthma are self-administering their inhaled medications incorrectly, according to a survey in the *Journal of General Internal Medicine*.

When the researchers asked 100 patients who were hospitalised for asthma or a lung disease to demonstrate how they used their inhalers, most of the patients did so incorrectly. They found roughly 90 percent of the study population misused their metered-dose inhalers, while the patients using Diskus inhalers made mistakes in 70 percent of their demonstrated efforts.

What is a nebuliser?

A nebuliser is operated by battery or A/C current that compresses air or oxygen to deliver a fine mist containing medication to the airways. There are three components: compressor, tubing and chamber with mask. Strictly speaking, the chamber nebulises the solution into airways; the air is compressed by the machine. Nebulisers are usually used to deliver reliever medications to the lung during asthma flare-ups. Many parents mistakenly believe that a nebuliser is a more efficient device than a spacer. In fact high doses of inhaled bronchodilator can be given via a large volume spacer that produces equivalent clinical effects to a nebuliser. In fact many children's emergency departments routinely use large volume spacers as opposed to nebulisers, in order to give reliever treatments in asthma attacks. Physicians do not routinely prescribe nebulisers because they are bulky, expensive and administration times are much longer. The noise of the compressor can frighten smaller children. They need to be serviced once each year and depending on the device, it may not be possible to use it without a transformer in Europe and the USA.

How do you use a nebuliser?

Wash your hands before handling the equipment or medication. Plug in the compressor. Most medications (Ventolin®, Atrovent®, Pulmicort®, Flixotide®) come in a premixed plastic vial; the cap is removed and the contents are emptied into the nebuliser chamber. Keep the chamber level and attach it and its tubing to the compressor. Fit the mask onto your child's face or put the mouthpiece into position, then switch on the device. A nebulisation typically lasts fifteen minutes. The treatment is finished when all of the treatment fluid has been removed. The nebuliser chamber and tubing should be washed daily in warm soapy water, then rinsed and allowed to air dry before re-use. Wipe your child's face and give them a drink after each nebuliser session.

> **What does 'adherence' mean?**

'Adherence' is a term to describe how compliant a patient is with their prescribed medication regime. It is well recognised by the medical profession that in chronic conditions like asthma not all patients take treatment as recommended all the time. There are many reasons for why this happens: sometimes it is lack of routine or time; sometimes it can be for financial reasons; sometimes it is because people don't understand why a treatment is necessary because it hasn't been properly explained by their doctor; and sometimes it is denial of the underlying condition – often seen with teenagers.

When children are symptomatic it is generally easy to remember to take medications, particularly one's reliever medication, which works quickly and provides almost instant feedback. However, once things have settled down and asthma has become quiescent, it can be difficult to remember to take preventative treatment. It must be remembered that it takes several weeks for inhaled steroids to start working and it can take many weeks for symptoms to reoccur if the inhaler is discontinued. Thus, there is no immediate negative or positive feedback perceived with controller treatment. Studies have consistently shown that inhaled steroids only control asthma as long as they are taken regularly and that the steroid effect wears off within three months. Inhaled steroids have no effect on the natural history of the condition; they simply suppress inflammation, which translates into a reduction of symptoms.

A common scenario occurs during the summer, when levels of viral infection within the community drops and children are out of school. Asthma undergoes a natural improvement and some parents will discontinue their child's preventative treatment thinking that they have outgrown the condition. When September arrives, they have been off treatment for two to three months, the protective effect of inhaled steroids has worn off, and on return to school there is a natural resurgence in viral activity, which occurs consistently each year in the thirty-sixth week, usually two weeks after starting back at school. When the child encounters their first head cold of the season, their asthma flares up again. It is vital for doctors prescribing preventative treatment to ensure that their patients (or their parents) understand the rationale for taking treatment and that it is not discontinued without input from the prescribing physician.

How do colds and flu affect asthma?

It is well recognised that viral upper respiratory infections frequently trigger asthma flare-ups in children. The asthmatic airway appears to be especially sensitive to rhino-viruses (cold viruses), of which there are many strains. These viruses are more prevalent in our winter months when children are at school and ambient temperatures drop.

In my practice parents often ask about the 'flu'. It must be remembered that influenza is just another respiratory virus that causes illness. Typical symptoms include fever, runny nose, cough, body aches and sore throat. It occurs as two forms: Influenza A and B, both of which can mutate (change genetic makeup) from year to year. Influenza A viruses are categorised into subtypes on the basis of two surface proteins, hemagglutinin and neur-aminidase. Influenza B undergoes less mutation than Influenza A, and is not categorised into subtypes. Influenza C causes only mild illness and is not categorised into subtypes. Wild birds naturally carry Influenza A, but don't normally become sick as a result of it. Domesticated birds, such as chickens, can become very sick as a result of Influenza A. Some subtypes of the Influenza A virus can infect both birds and humans — this is the major concern for avian flu or 'bird flu'. Pigs ('swine flu') can also be infected by Influenza A subtypes. These forms don't normally infect humans, but reports of animal to human transmission, and human to human transmission, have occurred. Normally, symptoms from influenza infection resolve without treatment in healthy people within a matter of days.

However, people with chronic heart and lung diseases, diabetes, the elderly, and young children are at risk of complications from influenza infection. Complications, including bacterial infections and pneumonia can occur, resulting in hospitalisation and even death, particularly within these high-risk groups. Influenza infections may cause worsening asthma symptoms. Complications from influenza infection are more common in asthmatics than in people without asthma, and may include severe asthma attacks, pneumonia, and may result in hospitalisation and rarely death if untreated.

The best way to treat influenza infection is to prevent it from occurring in the first place. Each year, a flu vaccine is produced against the most prevalent strains of influenza, and is recommended for children with high-risk medical conditions such as asthma. In the winter of 2009 – 10, the annual flu shot did not protect against H1N1 infection and supplementary vaccination was required. This vaccine has been shown to prevent or reduce the severity of infection as well as the complications from infection. Vaccination ought to be given annually in October, in order to provide protection against that year's influenza subtypes as well as to provide a boosting effect, as protection from the vaccine begins to fade after one year. In addition, good hygiene can be helpful in preventing influenza. Frequent hand washing or the use of alcohol-based hand cleaners can help prevent the transmission of the influenza virus. People with influenza infection should stay at home until they are deemed non-infectious. Despite these measures, some asthmatics will become infected with the flu. Medications are available for the treatment of influenza infections, which have been shown to reduce the severity and duration of symptoms when taken within forty-eight hours of the start of the illness.

Zanamavir and Oseltamivir are newer anti-viral medications that are effective for the treatment and prevention of infection from seasonal influenza and swine flu. Zanamavir (Relenza®) is an inhaled medication, while Oseltamivir (Tamiflu®) is an oral medication; both work by preventing the influenza virus from replicating inside the cells of a person's respiratory tract. In addition to anti-viral medications, worsening asthma symptoms during an influenza infection also need to be treated. When influenza infection results in worsening asthma symptoms, oral steroids and increased reliever inhalers may be needed. Occasionally, asthmatics who get the flu need to be hospitalised. Your child's regular controller therapy should also be continued during this time.

Do milk and dairy products produce mucus and make asthma worse?

Mucus is produced by cells within the nose, sinuses and lungs. It consists of water, salt and various proteins that help trap germs and particles of dirt. Antibacterial enzymes and proteins called antibodies in mucus also help to kill germs and protect from infection. Mucus is moved towards the back of the throat by microscopic hair cells called cilia, where it is then swallowed. Excessive mucus production occurs with viral URTI or nasal allergy, and may lead to a cough, sore throat and hoarseness. Sometimes nasal mucus can trickle down the back of the throat, leading to post-nasal drip. Thick, dry mucus can also irritate the throat and be hard to clear. Dry mucus is more common in older people and in dry inland climates. Air conditioning, winter heating, dehydration and some medications (such as some antihistamines, antidepressants and blood pressure medicines) can aggravate the condition. Some children notice that when they drink milk or other dairy products, their throat feels coated and mucus is thicker and harder to swallow. Recent research has shown that these sensations are due to the texture of the fluid and occur with similar liquids of the same thickness, and are not due to increased production of mucus. Symptoms of cow's milk allergy are very different and described elsewhere.

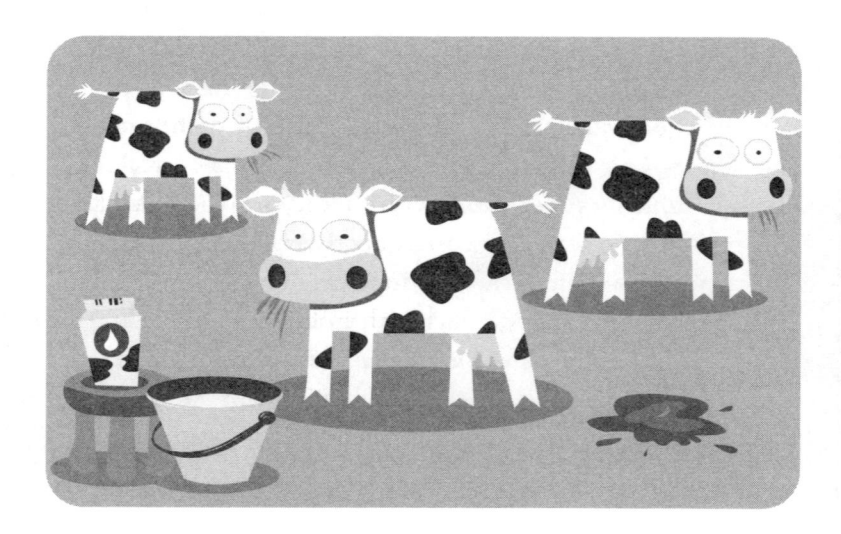

Middle ear infections are very common in early childhood. Infections are even more common when children also have allergic rhinitis (hay fever). Allergic inflammation causes swelling in the nose and around the opening of the Eustachian tube, interfering with drainage of the middle ear. Mucus may accumulate there (glue ear) and infection (otitis) can ensue. Children with cow's milk allergy sometimes appear to suffer from more frequent infections. This is not because milk causes infection, but rather because children with food allergy are more likely to suffer from other allergic disorders such as allergic rhinitis. Asthma and allergic rhinitis (hay fever) are normally triggered by substances that we inhale, such as pollen, dust mite, mould spores or animal dander. Dairy products rarely trigger asthma or allergic rhinitis. When they do, nasal symptoms are usually accompanied by obvious symptoms of allergy, such as severe hives, throat or tongue swelling or a drop in blood pressure. Recent studies have shown that milk has no effect on lung function, and does not trigger symptoms in patients with asthma any more than placebo. When patients complain of cough after having cold milk, it is usually due to breathing in cool air as they drink, and usually disappears if they warm the milk first. Some parents have already placed their child on a milk-free diet when they come to see me. Invariably it is of no benefit. Research has shown that eliminating dairy products from a diet does not improve asthma or rhinitis.

Of more concern is that the unnecessary elimination of milk products from a child's diet may adversely affect their nutrition. Milk and other dairy products are an important source of calcium and other minerals needed for strong teeth and growing bones. If there are proven medical reasons to exclude milk and other dairy products from your child's diet, it is important to ensure that you substitute other calcium-containing foods and drinks, or take a calcium supplement. It is often a good idea to consult a dietitian. The take-home message should be that in the vast majority of most sufferers, dietary restriction is of no benefit in asthma or allergic rhinitis, and distracts efforts away from more productive areas such as trigger and allergen avoidance.

> 'Our child has asthma. Our ENT surgeon says she has glue ear and wants to insert grommets shortly. Are general anaesthetics safe for children with asthma?'

Firstly, glue ear with hearing deficit is very common in children with allergies. These children frequently have regular nasal symptoms due to allergic rhinitis, which in turn causes Eustachian tube dysfunction and an accumulation of thick mucous in the middle ear leading to infections and hearing loss. As stated earlier in the book, nasal allergy co-exists with asthma in up to 50 percent of cases.

The most important thing for any asthmatic child undergoing a general anaesthetic is to ensure that their symptoms are properly controlled. This may require a pre-operative check-up with your GP or specialist. They will tell you whether your child's asthma is controlled and whether they are medically fit for the anaesthetic. Your child will be seen on the day of the procedure by your Consultant Anaesthetist who ought to have special expertise in dealing with children. They will ascertain whether or not your child is well on the day of surgery and that they have not recently contracted any common viral infection as this will lead to cancellation of the procedure on the day.

Many commonly used anaesthetic drugs produce bronchodilation and generally do not cause asthmatic children any trouble. In Ireland, thousands of asthmatic children have surgery under general anaesthesia every year without any ill effects.

What are dust mites?

Dust mite allergy is seen in as many as 80 percent of asthmatic children residing in temperate climates of developed countries. There appears to be a close relationship between dust sensitisation, asthma and allergic rhinitis. Often the allergy precedes the symptoms. Dust mites (*Dermatophagoides pteronyssinus*) are microscopic insects that feed on organic detritus such as flakes of shed human skin and thrive in the stable environment of dwell-ings. House dust mites are the most common allergen found in asthmatic children in developed countries. Some of their gut enzymes (notably proteases), which persist in their faecal matter, are strongly allergenic. The house dust mite can survive in all climates, even at high altitude, however they flourish in the warm and humid indoor environment provided by homes, especially during the winter months in temperate climates. Dust mites dwell in mattresses, carpets, furniture and bedding, at concentrations of 188 animals per gram of dust. Even in dry climates, house dust mites survive and reproduce easily in bedding (especially in pillows), deriving moisture from the humidity generated by human breathing, perspiration and saliva.

The following measures are recommended for children with asthma or allergic rhinitis who have documented dust-mite allergy. Bed linen should be washed weekly at 60 degrees Celsius. Dry cleaning and tumble-drying at 55 degrees Celsius is also effective. Mattresses, pillows and duvet covers manufactured from specialised fabrics, which form a barrier to dust mites, should be used. Sheer floor surfaces like wood or lino are preferable to carpets. Books, dolls, teddy bears and toys should be stowed away or removed from the bedroom because they all increase the surface area on which the dust can settle. If possible, bedrooms should be naturally ventilated frequently and exposed to as much sunlight as possible. This reduces the humidity and the UV light kills off moulds and fungi, which feed on discarded skin flakes. Several clinical trials have shown that dehumidification can inhibit the proliferation of dust mites; however, this does not always translate into a clinical effect, as studies addressing the question have yielded conflicting results.

At the time of writing, the use of a dehumidifier cannot be routinely recommended. However, there may be specific situations where the indoor environment is particularly humid or damp, and there may be an excess of fungal spores leading to poor respiratory health. Acaricides such as benzyl benzoate and tannic acid have been used to kill dust mites. Their use has been assessed in trials but their efficacy is as yet unproven. Some antidust fabrics have been impregnated with acaricides, which theoretically should amplify the effect. Devices have been developed for interrupting the growing cycle of dust mites (Drontech®). They act by transmitting pulsing ultrasonic waves at a frequency of 40,000 Hz, which is completely harmless to humans, but it is alleged these waves interfere with the lifecycle of house dust mites, thus reducing their concentration in the room that the device is used. However, to date there has been no study published in a peer-reviewed journal that supports their use.

A favourite cuddly toy should be put in the freezer and then vacuumed or if possible, put in a wash at 60 degrees Celsius. If dust avoidance is to succeed, children with a dust allergy should sleep in Spartan conditions. I tell parents that the bedroom should resemble a monk's cell (no carpet, a bed, a bedside locker and a book). Damp dusting, vacuuming and de-cluttering of the room needs to be performed on a regular basis each week. The effort needs to be consistent to achieve results; half measures will be ineffective.

There is some debate within the medical community as to whether these interventions are beneficial for asthma, based mainly on an analysis (Cochrane review) of published papers over the last thirty years. The data used was heterogeneous and consisted of often quite old papers of relatively poor quality, where effect of dust mite intervention was not evaluated by means of dust allergen assays. However, there have been a number of clinical studies where dust-allergic children were moved from high to low dust environments. After six months, the children all exhibited lower allergy reactions to dust mite, their pulmonary function had improved and medication requirements were reduced. Most clinicians who care for asthmatic patients and asthma advocacy groups across the globe continue to recommend dust-avoidance measures in patients with documented dust allergy.

> **My child has asthma. Can they have a pet?**

Not all children with asthma will have allergy to household pets and not all of those who are sensitised will have their symptoms exacerbated by the pet. However, animal allergens remain a potent trigger of both acute and chronic asthma symptoms. As many as 66 percent of asthmatic children will be sensitised to cat and dog dander. Indoor exposure to pet dander can adversely affect asthma control. Interestingly, studies have shown that many homes contain these allergens, even if the animal has not been resident there. Cat dander is very sticky and it is likely that children become sensitised indirectly by exposure to clothing, walls and carpets outside the home. Approximately 15 percent of these allergens are sufficiently small as to be airborne; naturally air samples from homes with cats will contain allergen but cat allergen can be found in air samples from homes without cats.

There have been far fewer trials addressing the efficacy of dander control measures compared to those looking at dust mites. Thus the following recommendations are predominantly opinion- rather than evidence-based. Removal of the source of the allergen is the first step. However, the beneficial effect of that intervention may take time to become apparent as it may take several months for allergen levels to decline. Levels of allergen may fall more rapidly if sources of the dander are removed, for example carpet. Aggressive cleaning of allergen reservoirs, animal sleeping cushions etc, may also enhance this effect. There is no convincing data suggesting that meaningful decreases in pet allergen concentrations can occur without removal of the animal from the home. Tannic acid has been shown to produce short-term reductions in allergen levels and may be useful if combined with removal of the offending pet. If a family wish to retain their pet, it should be restricted to one area within the home, and not allowed near the patient's bedroom. Consideration should be given to the installation of an air filtration, e.g. HEPA or electrostatic systems.

Horse hair may be quite allergenic and can cause a dramatic allergy reaction (anaphylaxis), including an asthma attack. Children with horse allergy should avoid any direct exposure to horses or their stables. Parents who ride or whose occupation involves regular horse exposure should note that the allergen may adhere to their clothing and contaminate their vehicle, and that these indirect exposures may be harmful.

> **Is dampness harmful to children with asthma?**

In normal circumstances, we all encounter moulds each day. People are routinely exposed to as many as two hundred different species. We regularly inhale spores and our immune system generally deals with them and they are eliminated. Some climates are more humid than others and atmospheric levels of mould will be higher in these areas. Damp, indoor living conditions can lead to the growth of moulds and fungi. They can be detected in air samples and damp patches and mildew are visible manifestations of the problem. Studies have shown that visible mould growth is associated with increase cough, phlegm production and bronchitis. Dampness occurs where there is inadequate ventilation or excessive moisture. Sometimes fungal spores of *Aspergillus fumigatus* can be released from old plasterwork during the renovation of houses. It is evident that damp accommodation can give rise to increased allergy-related symptoms and an increased rate of respiratory illness. The proposed mechanisms for these findings include allergic sensitisation to dust mite and moulds, immunosupression by fungal products, and irritant effects from volatile substances emitted by moulds. One study in mice showed that nasal inoculation with the fungi *Stachybotrys chartarum* caused bronchial inflammation and haemorrhage. Fungi produce mycotoxins, which can interfere with the function of macrophages and may lead to respiratory tract infection. One study in infants demonstrated that exposure to high levels of fungi at home during infancy increases the risk of respiratory infections. An extreme example of how fungi affects the lung is allergic broncopulmonary aspergillosis, which is a hypersensitivity reaction to the fungus *Aspergillus fumigatus*. It can arise *de novo*, or may sometimes complicate an underlying lung condition such as bronchiectasis, more severe forms of asthma and cystic fibrosis. It produces symptoms that are not dissimilar to asthma. Allergy tests to Aspergillus are strongly positive and total IgE is elevated. In contrast to asthma, Chest X-rays are abnormal and the condition is treated with oral steroids and antifungal medication.

If you have a problem with damp in your home or a particular bedroom, it is important that the source of the excess moisture be identified and fixed. The questions that need to be addressed are whether the room is correctly vented, and if there is a water leak. There are companies who can perform air sampling to measure moisture and fungal loads. They will often compare the indoor concentration of fungi to that measured outdoors. If a damp problem is identified then correct damp-coursing, repair of water leaks, optimisation of ventilation and dehumidification may solve the problem. This is especially true if one lives in basement accommodation or if a bedroom is specifically affected. In summary, damp housing conditions have an adverse effect on the respiratory health of your child and ought to be addressed before embarking on medical investigations and treatment.

> **Do household cleaning agents and sprays affect asthma?**

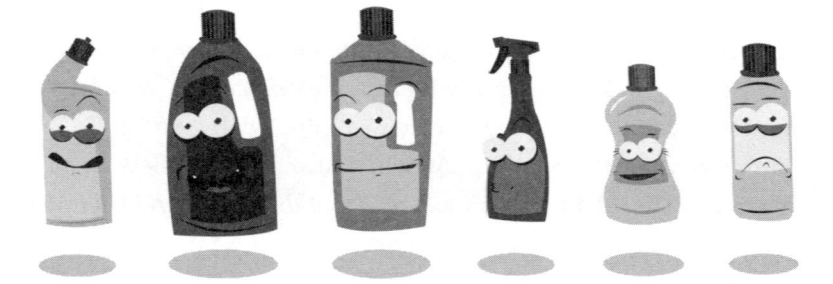

This question has been addressed by several studies in adults and the answer is most definitely yes. Professional domestic cleaners have a higher prevalence of asthma than the rest of the population. These products contain many chemicals, including alcohol, ammonia, chlorine-releasing substances, glycol ethers, sodium hydroxide, acryl polymers, terpenes and hypochlorite. There are reports of cross-contamination of bleaches, which contain ammonia, and other products containing hydrochloric acid. They combine to form trichloramine gas, which can induce asthma. A pivotal study regarding this was published in 2007, in which researchers investigated the risk of new-onset asthma over a nine-year period in relation to the use of common household cleaners. Using the European Community Respiratory Health Survey in ten countries, they identified 3,500 persons doing the cleaning in their homes who were free of asthma. Frequency of use of fifteen types of cleaning products was obtained in a face-to-face interview at follow-up. They subsequently studied the incidence of asthma (defined as physician diagnosis and as symptoms or asthma medication usage) at follow-up. They found that the use of cleaning sprays at least weekly was associated with a higher incidence of asthma symptoms or medication. The incidence of physician-diagnosed asthma was higher among those using sprays at least four days per week. The more sprays used, the higher the risk for asthma appeared to be. Risks were predominantly found for commonly used glass-cleaning, furniture, and air-refreshing sprays. Cleaning products in liquid or gel form were not associated with asthma.

Another study looking at chemical household product use and wheezing in preschool children was performed in the Avon region of the UK. The frequency of use of eleven chemical-based domestic cleaning products was determined by questionnaire. It was completed by women during pregnancy and a total chemical burden calculated. It was found was that frequent use of chemical-based products in the prenatal period is associated with persistent wheezing in young children. A follow up study of this cohort is underway.

> **How does environmental tobacco smoke affect asthma?**

Nowadays, everybody knows that they should not smoke and that if they can't break the habit, at the very least they should never smoke in a confined space like a car or indoors at home. We also know that the tobacco industry targets young people. Young people with asthma should never smoke and childhood is when 90 percent of current smokers became addicted. Tobacco smoke, whether inhaled directly or in the form of second-hand smoke, is dangerous to health. If you have asthma, it can make things even worse. Chronic obstructive pulmonary disease (COPD) affects older people who have smoked. This is often called chronic bronchitis or emphysema. There is an emerging link between smoking, childhood asthma and COPD in later life. Unlike asthma, treatments for COPD are not very effective because they cannot replace lost or damaged lung tissue. Second-hand smoke, also known as environmental tobacco smoke, is a combination of the smoke from a burning cigarette, cigar or pipe and the smoke exhaled from a smoker's lungs. Over four thousand different chemicals can be found in tobacco smoke. More than fifty of them are known or probable causes of cancer, and six are hazardous to growing children and unborn babies. Second-hand smoke contains: formaldehyde (embalming fluid), cyanide (poison), arsenic (poison), carbon monoxide (car exhaust), methane (poison), benzene (poison in cleaning solvent), nitro amines (cancer-causing compounds), cadmium (toxic metal), benzopyrene (cancer-causing substance found in gasoline and tar), aniline (poison used in dye) and polonium (radioactive materials). Children exposed to environmental tobacco smoke may develop more asthma and may have more frequent and severe asthma attacks. They are also at higher risk of getting pneumonia and bronchitis and having poorer lung function.

Children exposed to second-hand smoke are more likely to get more middle ear infections. Young infants exposed to tobacco smoke are at a higher risk for Sudden Infant Death Syndrome, which is the main cause of death in babies between one month and one year of age. We all know that mothers who smoke in pregnancy have more premature and low birth weight babies. Non-smoking partners of smokers should know that they are nearly five times more likely to develop asthma in adulthood than those who are not exposed to second-hand smoke. Non-smokers who are regularly exposed to second-hand smoke at home or work have almost double the risk of heart disease.

> **Are domestic gas fumes dangerous for children with asthma?**

All domestic gas appliances generate Nitrogen dioxide (NO2). Laboratory studies show that NO2 exposure in animals can increase allergic sensitisation to allergens. It has been shown in a study from Singapore that lung function drops in asthmatic females following acute exposure to gas from outdoor cooking on stoves. Other studies have shown that repeated exposures through cooking causes increased bronchodilator use among asthmatic females. Furthermore, an inverse correlation was demonstrated between NO2 levels and lung function in Australian school children. In other words, the higher the measured NO2, the lower the level of lung function. In a prospective study of 728 asthmatic children, regular home NO2 measurements were taken. Those who cooked with an electric stove had an average NO2 reading of 8.6ppb, whereas those who cooked with gas had an average of 25.9ppb. The authors noted that there were increased asthma symptoms with levels below the US Environmental Protection Agency outdoor threshold of 58ppb. Most authorities would agree that high NO2 levels may induce asthma in susceptible individuals but probably do not cause it. The risk of exposure is highest where multiple families share a dwelling and where gas appliances are unvented.

> **Can air filters help prevent asthma symptoms?**

Room air cleaners remove small particles that are in the air near the air cleaner. However, room air cleaners do not remove small allergen particles that are caused by local disturbances, such as the microscopic house dust mite faeces that surround a pillow when your head hits it (or you turn over in bed). You inhale these allergens before they ever get near the room air cleaner. Room air cleaners take five to fifteen minutes to remove such temporary local sources of dust and allergens. Wall-to-wall carpets also provide a large source of dust mite allergens (100,000 dust mites lives in 1 square metre of carpet). They simply cannot be removed by vacuuming or the use of a room air cleaner. However, these accumulated allergens remain in the carpet until disturbed. Vacuuming carpets, which uses a beater brush, causes very large amounts of allergens to be thrown into the room air, even if a HEPA vacuum cleaner is used. Thus the dust should be allowed to settle for several hours prior to the child sleeping in the room. Room air cleaners only work for the room in which they are placed. Since a child may spend ten to twelve hours in the bedroom every night, that's logically the first room in which to locate a room air cleaner. At the time of writing, room filtration systems cannot be recommended for the routine management of asthma. They may be an option in particular situations where there are unavoidably high levels of indoor allergens and tobacco smoke.

How do rhinitis and sinusitis diseases relate to asthma?

For some time now, the nasal passages and bronchial tubes have been viewed as a continuum of the same system. This concept, known as the united airway or single airway theory, acknowledges that inflammation in one region can have an adverse effect in the other. Research indicates that at least 50 percent of children with asthma have co-existing allergic rhinitis. Many more asthmatics will also get hay fever. Allergic nasal disease is under-diagnosed and undertreated in children. In my experience, children rarely complain of nasal symptoms because they have become accustomed to them over a long period of time. Seasonal allergic rhinitis can co-exist with a chronic allergic rhinitis. The house dust mite is a key driver of allergic rhinitis whereas grass pollen is the main trigger for hay fever, which presents more acute and noticeable symptoms. Untreated or undertreated nasal allergy can lead to chronic sinus infection. The paranasal sinuses are a series of air-filled cavities located in the bones around the midface. The entrance into the sinus system occurs through a narrow orifice in the nasal passages called the sinus ostium. If the nasal lining becomes inflamed, this ostium becomes blocked and mucus can accumulate within the sinus system, which can become infected. Infants and toddlers do not get sinus infections because the sinuses only start to develop between five to eight years of age, thus sinusitis generally only occurs in older school-going children.

When infected sinus secretions are inhaled into the lower airways during sleep, chest infections can ensue. Even uncomplicated nasal allergy can lead to poor asthma control and an increased requirement for asthma medications. The mechanisms for this phenomenon are not proven but may involve the sino-bronchial reflex (where inflammation of the sinus provokes spasm of the lower airways), aspiration of infected sinus secretions and systemic release of inflammatory mediators. It is vital that every patient being assessed for asthma also be evaluated specifically for symptoms and signs of allergic rhinitis. The patient should also have a complete ENT examination specifically evaluating the patient for the presence of allergic rhinitis.

Typical symptoms of allergic rhinitis consist of nasal congestion, clear nasal secretions, sneezing (typically first thing in the morning), a constant clearing of the throat and a regular rubbing of the nose. Physical findings consist of a pale and swollen lining of the nasal passages, reduced flow through the nasal passages and a transverse nasal crease from constant rubbing. Older children and adults may develop nasal polyps. Treatment of allergic rhinitis can improve asthma control without any change to therapy for asthma. Treatment consists of allergen avoidance, antihistamines and topical nasal steroids in the first instance. Any concurrent sinus infection needs to be treated and will frequently require quite protracted courses of antibiotics for up to four weeks. Other treatments may be required to treat more complicated cases. Sometimes a sinus CT scan will be necessary and very occasionally an ENT surgeon may need to perform functional endoscopic sinus surgery (FESS). There is a reluctance to do so in children because of the potential effect on the development of the mid-facial bones. The relationship between asthma and allergic rhinitis has been recognised by the ARIA guidelines.

> **Are salt caves (speleotherapy) helpful?**

There are records of improvements in the breathing of miners in Roman and medieval times. Dr Feliks Boczkowski – a physician at the Polish salt mine at Wieliczka – wrote in 1843 that the miners there did not suffer from lung diseases and his successor set up a spa based upon these observations. Modern use of this therapy started in Germany when Dr Karl Hermann Spannagel noticed improvement in the health of his patients after they hid in the Kluterthöhle karst cave to escape heavy bombing during World War II. It is now practised in places such as Slovakia, Wieliczka in Poland and in Ukraine. Much of the published data is in Russian.

Commercial salt cave clinics have been established elsewhere and have claimed excellent results. However, a Cochrane review group searched all the major medical-bioscientific electronic databases (Medline, Embase, Cochrane Airways group database), contacted speleotherapy centres and experts in the field, hand searched proceedings, and checked bibliographies of articles obtained to identify possible relevant publications. They included controlled clinical trials (i.e. both randomised and those not reporting the method of allocation) that compared clinical effects of speleotherapy with another intervention or no intervention in patients with chronic asthma. Information concerning patients, interventions, results and methodology were extracted in a standardised manner by two independent reviewers and summarised descriptively. Only 3 clinical trials, including a total of 124 asthmatic children, met the inclusion criteria, but only one trial had reasonable method-ological quality. Two trials reported that speleotherapy had a beneficial short-term effect on lung function. Other outcomes could not be assessed in a reliable manner. The reviewers concluded that the available evidence did not permit any reliable conclusion as to whether speleotherapeutic interventions are effective for the treatment of chronic asthma and that properly designed randomised controlled trials with long-term follow-up were needed.

> **What are Buteyko exercises?**

Buteyko is a form of physical therapy used for the treatment of asthma. The method takes its name from the late Ukrainian doctor Konstantin Pavlovich Buteyko, who first formulated its principles in the 1960s. At the core of the Buteyko method is a series of reduced-breathing exercises that focus on nasal-breathing, breath-holding and relaxation. It involves the taping of the mouth at night to encourage nasal-breathing. A recent study which addressed this particular intervention concluded that mouth-taping did not improve asthma control. It is certainly not recommended for children. Buteyko's theory was that asthmatics 'chronically overbreathe' and the exercises are designed to teach asthmatics to breathe less. The goal is to retrain breathing to a normal pattern, akin to certain forms of Yoga. The basic premise of Buteyko is that asthma is caused by an abnormal pattern of breathing condition called hyperventilation (rapid shallow breathing). We now know that this is not the case. However, breathing patterns may become dysfunctional as the result of chronic asthma in adults. This method, along with other types of breathing exercises, may be of benefit to certain subsets of asthma sufferers. In several clinical trials in adults, Buteyko has been shown to safely reduce asthma symptoms and the need for rescue medication, and in one study it resulted in a decreased requirement for inhaled corticosteroids. It does not seem to improve bronchial hyper-responsiveness or lung function. The method requires time and commitment and involves daily exercises over a period of weeks or months. There have been no satisfactory clinical trials specifically addressing its safety or efficacy in children.

> **What is bronchiolitis? Is it linked to asthma?**

Bronchiolitis describes a single episode of viral infection of the lower airways of infants (less than one year of age) typically caused by the respiratory syncitial virus (RSV), which is prevalent during the winter months. Some doctors mistakenly label recurrently wheezy infants as having bronchiolitis. In most cases, the infection with RSV is mild, producing a bad cold or upper respiratory tract infection. In fact, most infants will have encountered this infection by their second birthday. However, in 1 percent of cases, infants will require hospitalisation. They will be chesty, wheezy and off their feeds. Their breathing may be rapid and they may need oxygen. The RSV virus can be recovered from their nasal secretions in a rapid diagnostic test. Hospitalised infants are frequently younger, may have a history of premature delivery or be born to mothers who smoked during pregnancy. Other susceptible infants include those with underlying problems with lung disease, heart disease or defects of their immune system. Studies have shown that infants with a high risk of developing asthma are hosptalised with bronchiolitis.

> **My baby is wheezy. Do they have asthma?**

The short answer is probably not. Many babies will wheeze, but only a small proportion will become asthmatic. Many toddlers will wheeze only with a viral URTI and will not have an allergy history. This group of wheezers tends to settle by school age. We know a lot about the various types of asthma and their natural history from information gleaned from the Tucson Birth Cohort. Respiratory symptoms, allergy status and lung function was collected serially in a cohort of 1,200 children born during 1980 to 1984 in Tucson, Arizona and were followed from birth to the present day. The study showed how gender, birth weight and maternal antenatal smoking history influence lung function later in life. The cohort study also showed that some infants have only transient wheezing, which relates to initial abnormal lung function and which settles by school age. Other infants have what is termed persistent wheeze, i.e. the tendency to wheeze persists throughout childhood, which was associated with a deterioration in lung function from initially normal levels. This is the group who have a clear history of atopy and are probably what we understand as asthmatics. Another group identified by the study were late onset wheezers who have normal lung function and who were asymptomatic during infancy.

> **When I was pregnant I threatened to go into early labour. The doctors gave me a steroid injection to help my babies lungs mature. Could this have caused their asthma?**

I am sometimes asked whether antenatal steroids given to mothers at risk of premature labour are harmful to babies. Premature babies have less well developed airways, which have a narrower calibre. These infants are more prone to wheezing illness in the first year of life. Most of these infants will not evolve into asthmatics. There have been a number of studies which addressed the question of whether antenatal steroids protect against asthma in later life. Three studies showed no effect. One study showed a higher risk of asthma and two showed a protective effect against the development of asthma. None of the studies were of sufficiently robust design to rely solely on their result. At the time of writing, I would argue that antenatal steroids do not have harmful effects on the infant lung and that they do not predispose to asthma later in life.

What are allergy tests?

Allergy tests can be done on the skin (skin prick test) or blood (a specific IgE or RAST test). Both are scientifically proven to detect allergy. Skin tests are more sensitive, i.e will detect more allergies, and have the advantage of providing results immediately. Skin tests detect more allergies if performed on the back, particularly the upper back, rather than the arm. RAST tests require a blood draw and there is a delay whilst the laboratory processes the sample. Subjects must refrain from taking antihistamines for twenty–four to seventy–two hours prior to a skin test. This restriction does not apply to a RAST test.

Skin prick tests are performed by a physician, nurse or technician. These are performed on the forearm or back by means of a lancet and a series of allergens (food and/or inhalants). Histamine and saline are used as positive and negative controls. Allergen drops are placed on a grid that is drawn on the skin, and the lancet is used to introduce the substance into the dermis or supeficial layer. If an allergy is present a small hive will develop and its size measured after fifteen minutes. The test is safe. Side effects include a large local reaction and it has been reported that rarely a severe generalised reaction (anaphylaxis) can occur – in approximately 15 cases per 100,000 tests. I have never observed a severe generalised reaction to skin prick tests in over twenty years of practice. However, adrenalin and antihistamine should always be on hand. Unproven or unscientific allergy tests include kinesiology, leucocytotoxic test, electrodermal (Vega) test, hair analysis, iridology and pulse test

In February 2011, the UK's National Institute of Clinical Excellence (NICE) produced guidelines for allergy testing in children, what follows are excerpts from their press release:

Children are being placed on restrictive and potentially dangerous diets as parents look to the internet and the high street for alternative tests to diagnose food allergy, NICE warns. NICE has issued the first ever national guideline on food allergy in children which advises against the use of alternative tests, such as Vega testing, hair analysis and kinesiology.

The use of these alternative tests is on the increase because of a lack of allergy services on the NHS and difficulties with diagnosing the condition in primary care. But there is very little evidence to support the use of these unscientific tests, some of which can retail for £60 or more. It is estimated that of those children who report an allergy, 20 percent wrongly self-report diagnoses of various food allergies and do not eat certain foods because they think they are allergic to them.

NICE recommends that GPs, practice nurses and health visitors diagnose and assess a suspected food allergy, commonly an allergy to cow's milk, fish and shellfish or peanuts, using either skin prick testing or by taking a blood test for IgE antibodies.

This decision should be based on the results of the allergy-focused clinical history and whether the test is suitable, safe and acceptable to the child.

Dr Adam Fox, Consultant in Paediatric Allergy at Guys and St Thomas' Hospital in London who was involved in the development of the NICE guideline, said: "These are the only two scientifically proven tests that should be carried out to diagnose food allergy, and they should be validated alongside a full clinical history".

"It is very frustrating when you see a patient who has had a bad deal. Parents often think that these alternative tests offer a quick fix but many children often end up on restrictive diets".

> **What are pulmonary function tests (PFTs)?**

PFTs are a group of procedures that measure the function of the lungs and may provide the diagnosis in many common lung conditions. Individuals with chronic cough, breathlessness, wheeze and exercise induced symptoms may benefit from these tests. They can be used to confirm the diagnosis and track the progress of the following disorders: asthma, chronic bronchitis (bronchiectasis, cystic fibrosis and pulmonary fibrosis. PFTs enable clinicians to assess an individual's response to a given therapy. They are frequently requested by anaesthetists as part of a pre-operative assessment of individuals undergoing major surgery and may also be used in healthy individuals who undergo routine health-checks and for those undergoing pre-employment screening. Tests are usually done in a doctor's office or hospital clinic. Patients should refrain from taking bronchodilator medications, which can affect the result of the test. The subject wears a nose clip and performs a series of forced exhalations under the instruction of a pulmonary function technician. The tests are easy to perform, safe and well tolerated. Children as young as four years can co-operate with the technician. The problem in asthma is narrow bronchial tubes leading to delayed lung emptying, which is represented by an obstructive pattern on a pulmonary function test. A bronchodilator can be given to correct the situation. If the improvement is greater than 12 percent it is possible to diagnose asthma. Normal tests and the absence of a bronchodilator response do not rule out asthma and it is sometimes necessary to perform a bronchial provocation test. Results are generated by a computer programme and are expressed as a percent predicted for age, sex, race and height. It is important that a pulmonary specialist review the result and issue an official report.

Bronchial provocation tests are more detailed pulmonary function tests done in people with normal pulmonary function test results (without a bronchodilator response) where there is a suspicion of asthma or where asthma needs to be excluded.

There are many types of tests. The most commonly performed in this country uses methacholine, histamine, mannitol or exercise. These tests are generally performed in a hospital by a respiratory technician with a physician available. The aim of the test is to produce a 20 percent drop in lung function, which is diagnostic of asthma. These tests involve either a series of inhalations or exercising on a treadmill after which a series of measurements of lung function are made. Generally these tests are safe once performed on the right sort of patient in the correct setting. There is the potential to provoke an asthma attack; however, the drops in lung function are usually small enough not to cause any major symptoms. Any drops in lung function are corrected using inhaled bronchodilator. Another available test is exhaled nitric oxide (eNO), which can be measured in breath for asthma or other conditions characterised by airway inflammation.

What is exhaled NO?

NO stands for nitric oxide, a gas that is produced by the cells that line the inner wall of the airways and must be distinguished from Nitrogen dioxide (NO_2) which is an air pollutant. When the airways are inflamed, there are more eosinophils present, which release more NO than normal.

The amount of NO in the air breathed out (exhaled) can be measured and may show how much inflammation there is in the lungs. In other words, a high level of NO means inflammation is present. Some experts believe that exhaled NO measurement offers clinicians a new method of diagnosing asthma and assessing patients' response to treatment, allowing clinician to step-up or down treatment more easily. Some studies have shown that with the combination of NO levels and clinical routine assessments, patients with asthma can achieve control with the reduced doses of inhaled corticosteroids. Exhaled NO is more closely linked to the allergic form of asthma, and not all patients with asthma have elevated NO levels. Some people believe that high or increasing levels can predict an asthma attack well before symptoms develop. But like many tests in asthma, it has its limitations. We have been using it in our asthma clinic for many years now and it has been useful in some – but not all – patients. A biomarker like this would be a very useful tool for managing asthma, however more research needs to be done in children to determine its utility in real life.

> **Are asthma medications dangerous? Do they cause dependency?**

Asthma drugs do not cause dependency. Relievers may be habitually overused, but they do not cause physical or psychological dependency. Asthma medications have a very safe track record compared to other medications, whether prescribed or those available 'over the counter'. The reality is that all medications have potential side effects. Regulations for the licensing of new drugs are very strict. Not only does the drug have to have an acceptable safety profile, but it must also be of proven clinical benefit in an appropriate group of disease sufferers. New drugs have to undergo several large clinical trials, often involving thousands of patients from many countries. A side effect profile will emerge, some effects will be non-specific like headache, nausea, tummy upset, diarrhoea, rash and will be common to many drugs

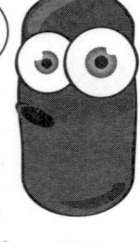

> Regulations for the licensing of new drugs are very strict

and often do not occur in excess when compared to placebo patients from the drug trial. Anaphylaxis can occur with any drug; aspirin, which is available over the counter, is associated with this. Some drugs can cause mild abnormality of heart, kidney or liver function. These effects can be monitored by the prescribing physician. Some people develop adverse reactions because of interactions with other drugs causing toxic blood levels.

Older or less frequently used drugs

Theophyllines

Theophyllines are members of the xanthine family and bear close structural similarity to caffeine. They occur naturally in tea and coffee, although in substantially less quantities than doses required for treatment. The potential benefits of coffee were first observed by the physician Sir John Floyers in the eighteenth century, who believed it helped his own asthma. Theophylline, also known as dimethylxanthine, is a methylxanthine drug used in therapy for respiratory diseases such as COPD or asthma under a variety of brand names. If blood levels become too high, children develop seizures and rhythm disturbances of the heartbeat. They are frequently taken orally, in a long-acting preparation, or given by injection. The intravenous form is reserved for very severe attacks of asthma where the child may be at risk of requiring intensive care and mechanical ventilation. Due to its numerous side-effects, such as nausea, vomiting, disturbance of sleep and hyperactive behaviour, these drugs are now rarely prescribed for children. The main benefits of theophylline in asthma are relaxing bronchial smooth muscle and possibly some anti-inflammatory effects, although these have yet to be satisfactorily confirmed to be clinically beneficial.

Cromolyn

Cromolyn sodium was discovered by Dr Roger Altounyan who was himself a lifelong asthma sufferer. It was considered a breakthrough drug in the management of asthma, mainly effective as a prophylaxis for allergic and exercise-induced asthma. Dr Altounyan had been evaluating certain medicinal plants with bronchodilating properties. One such plant was Khella (*Ammi visnaga*), which had been used as a muscle relaxant since ancient times in Egypt. Dr Altounyan deliberately inhaled derivatives of the active ingredient khellin to determine if they could prevent his asthma attacks. He eventually isolated an effective and safe asthma-preventing compound called cromolyn sodium. This drug prevents the release of inflammatory chemicals such as histamine from mast cells. Inhaled and topical preparations are available for allergic diseases of the lung, eye and nose (Intal®, Rhinocrom® and Opticrom®). This class of drug is no longer regularly prescribed for asthma in children, though it is still mentioned in treatment guidelines. Although it is free of major side effects, its relative lack of efficacy compared to inhaled steroids and onerous dosing regimen (four times daily) have lead to it being abandoned by most prescribers. It has been superseded by the antileukotriene class of drugs.

The underlying mechanism of action is not fully understood; while cromoglycate stabilises mast cells, this mechanism is probably not why it works in asthma. Pharmaceutical companies have produced twenty related compounds that are equally or more potent at stabilising mast cells and none of them have shown any anti-asthmatic effect. It is more likely that these work by inhibiting the response of sensory nerve fibres to the irritant capsaicin, inhibiting local axon reflexes involved in asthma, and may inhibit the release of T cell cytokines and mediators involved in asthma.

Newer and more regularly prescribed drugs

Antileukotrienes

The name leukotriene, introduced by Swedish biochemist Bengt Samuelsson in 1979, comes from the words leukocyte and triene. What would be later named leukotriene C, 'slow release substance of anaphylaxis' (SRS), was originally described between 1938 and 1940 by Feldberg and Kellaway. The researchers isolated SRS from lung tissue after a prolonged period following exposure to snake venom and histamine. Samuelsson subsequently received a Nobel Prize for Medicine. These substances are potent bronchoconstrictors and can cause inflammation of the lining tissue of the respiratory tract from the nose downwards. Antileukotriene drugs are the most commonly prescribed non-steroidal controller medications in children. They block the action of cysteinyl leukotrienes (e.g Montelukast®, Zafirlukast®) or prevent the production of leukotrienes (Zileuton®). First licensed in 1998, these drugs may be very effective in controlling asthma in some patients, but may have no therapeutic effect in others. Leukotriene inhibitors are generally more variable in their clincial efficacy than corticosteroids, but have virtually no serious side effects, so they are often used to treat children. They have a specific role for children where exercise-related symptoms are prominent.

Montelukast (Singulair®) is the most commonly prescribed antileukotiene drug worldwide. In contrast to most other asthma treatment, they are taken orally in the form of a chewable tablet or granules. There is no apparent method to determine who will or will not respond. Most clinicians would prescribe an eight-week trial. Most dramatic responses come within the first days or week of starting the medication.

The most common side effects with montelukast are headache, dizziness, abdominal pain, sore throat, and rhinitis (inflammation of the inner lining of the nose). These side effects occur in 1 in 100 to 1 in 10 persons who take montelukast. Rarely, patients may experience nose bleeds. Other side effects include hypersensitivity reactions, sleep disorders, nightmares and increased bleeding tendency, aside from many other generic adverse reactions like headache, nausea and gastrointestinal disturbance. Its use is associated with a higher incidence of Churg-Strauss syndrome (this probably relates to an 'unmasking' undiagnosed or subclinical Churg-Strauss). Most reports occurred initially with Zafirlukast (Accolate®) but it has also been linked to Montelukast (Singulair®). It must be stressed that a causal relationship between the antileukotriene drugs and Churg-Strauss Syndrome has not been established. In March 2008 the FDA announced that it would investigate whether mood changes and suicidal thoughts are possible side effects of drugs in this class, including the popular drug Singulair®, which currently lists these side effects.

On 12 June 2009, the Food and Drug Administration concluded their review into the possibility of neuropsychiatric side effects with leukotriene modulator drugs. Although clinical trials only revealed an increased risk of insomnia, post-marketing surveillance showed that the drugs are associated with a possible increase in suicidal behaviour and other side effects such as agitation, aggression, anxiousness, dream abnormalities and hallucinations, depression, irritability, restlessness and tremor. No firm evidence exists linking these possible psychiatric side effects to this class of drug, and this information shouldn't deter clinicians from prescribing them to children with asthma where appropriate.

Short-acting bronchodilators

For treating asthma symptoms in children there are two major types of short-acting bronchodilators: beta-agonists and anticholinergics. Depending on the drug, they are available in inhaled, tablet, liquid, and injectable forms. The preferred method of taking the beta-agonists and anticholinergics is by inhalation. Inhaled beta-agonists are by far the most commonly prescribed.

Short-acting bronchodilators, e.g. Salbutamol (Ventolin®) or Terbutaline (Bricanyl®), are rapidly-acting and are known as 'reliever' or 'rescue' medications. These bronchodilators relieve symptoms quickly by opening the airways. There can often be an immediate improvement, but they have no long-term effects on the condition. The rescue medications are best for treating sudden asthma symptoms. The action of inhaled bronchodilators starts within minutes after inhalation and lasts for two to four hours. Bronchodilators in asthma inhalers are also used fifteen to twenty minutes before exercise to prevent exercise-induced asthma. Short-acting bronchodilators can be used in an asthma nebuliser (breathing machine) to treat an asthma attack at home.

Oral forms of bronchodilators are usually reserved for toddlers who refuse to use a spacing device. When compared to inhalers, they tend to have more side effects because they are given in higher doses and have to travel throughout the bloodstream to get to the lungs. Whereas bronchodilators delivered by inhaler go directly into the lung and have fewer side effects because the dose is much lower. Overuse of short-acting bronchodilators is a sign of uncontrolled asthma that needs additional treatment. Asthma treatment guidelines suggest that, if your child is using their short-acting bronchodilators more than twice a week, you should visit your doctor to review your child's asthma controller therapy.

Side effects of beta-agonist bronchodilators include transient increases in pulse rate, tremor of the hands, behavourial disturbance and low blood potassium. These are more frequent with oral and IV formulations. Side effects of the antichloinergics like ipratropium bromide (Atrovent®) include dry mouth and transient increases in the heart rate.

> **Are inhaled corticosteroids dangerous? Do they suppress growth?**

Corticosteroids are powerful anti-inflammatory medications. They are sometimes confused with anabolic steroids, which are used illicitly by athletes to promote muscle development. Inhaled steroids are the most commonly prescribed preventative/controller medication for asthma. Older inhaled corticosteroids such as beclomethasone (e.g. Becotide, Beclazone) are topically less potent than the newer generation of inhaled steroids when delivered with standard inhalers. Some have been reformulated in an inhaler using very fine sprays (e.g. QVAR), which deliver the agents deep into the lungs and may prove to be as effective as the newer, more potent steroids. The swallowed dose of these medications has biological activity. Therefore, there is the potential for systemic side effects when used at high dose.

Newer generations of inhaled steroids include: fluticasone (Flixotide®); budesonide (Pulmicort®); triamcinolone (Azmacort®) and others. In general, the newer agents are topically more effective than the older generation of inhaled agents, and the swallowed dose is not biologically active. Treatment for more severe forms of asthma includes inhalers that combine both long-acting beta2-agonists and corticosteroids.

Side effects of inhaled steroids are surprisingly rare but include the following:

※ Throat irritation, hoarseness and dry mouth — effects which can be minimised by using a spacer device and rinsing the mouth after each treatment.

※ Allergy rashes, wheezing, facial swelling (oedema), fungal infections (thrush) in the mouth and throat, and bruising are also possible but are not common.

※ Hoarseness.

※ Very occasionally, a child can be exceptionally sensitive to the inhaled steroids and develop symptoms more commonly seen with oral steroids. They may experience changes in mood, memory, and behaviour — effects which can eliminated by reducing the dose.

※ Growth: it is comforting to know that when used in recommended doses, a number of studies report normal adult height is attained in children treated with inhaled steroids. Some studies show an initial deceleration in growth rate with beclomethasone (1-1.5cm) occurring within the first three months of treatment. Thereafter, growth velocity was normal. Again, the CAMP cohort study has yielded further data on final adult height. Analysis of the effects of inhaled steroids on height by age twenty in males and eighteen in females showed an overall effect of -1.2cm in final adult height versus those who did not receive inhaled steroids. Females were more markedly affected with -1.8cm compared to males at -0.8cm. Younger age at time of symptom onset and dose of inhaled steroid per body weight were associated with larger deficits. They concluded that reductions in growth occur shortly after inhaled steroid initiation are not cumulative but do persist into final adult height. Female gender and dose of steroid appear to have a greater influence on this initial effect and that the lowest effective dose should be used at treatment initiation. Growth suppressant effects of inhaled steroids were not apparent during the pubertal growth spurt.

✳ There is also some concern that the more potent agents, particularly fluticasone, suppress the adrenal system to a greater degree than other steroid inhalants. This effect in turn reduces levels of natural steroids — notably cortisol, the major stress hormone. (This is a serious side effect of oral steroids.) Of note, sudden changes in consciousness may suggest hypoglycemia, which can occur with adrenal insufficiency and was reported in a few children taking high doses of fluticasone. A 2002 study also observed abnormally low morning levels of cortisol in children taking fluticasone. It is believed that fluticazone was absorbed into the systematic blood stream via the lung. The swallowed dose becomes inactivated once absorbed from the stomach and it passes from the liver to the portal vein. A UK audit of those who developed serious side effects found that many of the children did not have asthma and others were on inappropriately high doses to control reasonably mild disease. It has been well established that long-term oral steroids or frequent bursts of oral steroids have a negative effect on bone density. It is not clear what effect long-term treatment with inhaled corticosteroid has; effects are likely to be dose-related. A Finnish study of 150 children published in 2010 found that, compared to cromolyn, regular inhaledsteroid treatment resulted in a significantly smaller increase in bone mineral density (0.023 versus 0.034 g/cm; p = 0.023) and height (7.75 versus 8.80 cm; p = 0.001) over eighteen months. However, height correlates closely with bone density.

* The CAMP study in the US looked at 1,000 children over seven years and initially reported that multiple oral corticosteroid bursts over a period of years can produce a dosage-dependent reduction in bone mineral accretion and increased risk for reduced bone density in children with asthma. However, bone density is correlated directly to height and it reflects skeletal maturity, pubertal status and physical activity. The CAMP investigators concluded that inhaled corticosteroid use has the potential for reducing bone mineral accretion in male children progressing through puberty, but this risk is likely to be outweighed by the ability to reduce the amount of oral corticosteroids used in these children. However, in the longer term follow-up of CAMP patients into early adulthood, no such effect was apparent in the cohort.

* Eye problems such as cataracts and glaucoma have been observed in adults receiving inhaled and oral steroids. This has not been found to be a problem with inhaled steroids in the few published paediatric studies.

Because the newer steroid inhalers, particularly fluticasone, may produce systemic side effects similar to oral steroids, it is important to aim for the lowest effective dose possible. Most studies suggest that low to moderate doses of inhaled steroids may achieve the same benefits as high doses, thus reducing risks for serious side effects. Better delivery methods may also allow lower doses.

Oral steroids

Oral corticosteroids are usually the last drugs to be added to an asthma treatment regime and the first to be removed. Common oral corticosteroids include prednisone/prednisolone, dexamethasone and methylprednisolone. They reduce inflammation very effectively, but children generally take them only for three to five days for an acute attack. Some children may find it hard to take them because they may have a bitter taste and can cause vomiting. Short courses of oral steroids are considered safe and are generally well tolerated by children. However, they can cause hyperactive behaviour, increase appetite and interfere with sleep. Prolonged use of oral steroids has widespread and sometimes serious side effects, and so they are not generally given to children for longer than a few days. Prolonged treatment with oral steroids causes serious side effects including supression of the adrenal gland, catarracts, osteoporosis, diabetes mellitus, weight gain, muscle wasting and depression. If someone on oral steroids develops chickenpox, they can get a more severe form if they have not been previously exposed or been vaccinated.

Long-acting beta-agonists (LABA)

Long-acting beta-agonists have been a recurring media focus since 2003, when the SMART study (Salmeterol Multicenter Asthma Research Trial) was halted early when a trend of worsening asthma and increased mortality (especially in African-Americans) was observed in patients on salmeterol compared to placebo. In addition, it didn't appear that the target enrolment of 60,000 study patients was going to be reached. Since that time, a plethora of opinions have been published, many of which suggest results of the SMART study do not reflect the outcomes of studies with combination LABA/steroid inhalers.

Post analysis of SMART showed that the African-American and Hispanic participants had more severe asthma (compared to Caucasians) at the start of the study. The SMART study was not solely used as a basis for subsequent black box warnings, but the data from it formed the backbone for the FDA proceedings.

In 2010, the FDA finalised new warnings for inhaled asthma drugs known as long-acting beta-agonists, exercising new powers to order the changes on products made by GlaxoSmithKline and AstraZeneca. The agency said it was requiring manufacturers to revise their labels because of an increased risk of severe exacerbation of asthma symptoms — and even death — in some patients using LABAs for the treatment of asthma.

The updated labels will now include language stating that the use of a LABA *without use of a long-term asthma control medication, such as an inhaled corticosteroid,* is not to be prescribed for the treatment of asthma. It also states that the products shouldn't be used in patients whose asthma is adequately controlled on low or medium dose inhaled corticosteroids. Serevent® and Foradil® contain only LABA, whereas Symbicort® and Seretide® contain a LABA and inhaled steroid. The safety findings in patients on LABA have been reproduced in the UK. It is postulated that mono-therapy with LABA, genetic polymorphisms of the 2-

receptor and racial differences in how these drugs are metabolised may explain this effect. In fact, several prospective studies addressing the genetic variations of the -receptor subunit have shown no correlation between the bronchodilator and bronchoprotective effects and genotype.

The best piece of work was conducted by the FDA themselves, who performed a meta-analysis of 60,000 patients and included data on all the pharmaceutical companies who produced LABA alone or in combination. In their analysis they showed a definite increased risk of death or adverse event from asthma in those patients on LABA inhalers not in combination with an inhaled steroid. However, when they looked at those on LABA in combination with an inhaled steroid the risk for death or adverse event dropped considerably to a level that does not appear significant. Yet, they recommended the cautious use of this class of drug and recommended optimising the dose of inhaled steroid when commencing this class of drug. I suspect that the adverse outcomes observed with the LABA inhaler relate to poorer compliance with inhaled steroids, leading to unrecognised inflammation and a masking of symptoms by the prolonged bronchodilator effect. It is my experience that this class of drug, when used in combination with an inhaled steroid, is very beneficial for the majority of patients with poorly controlled asthma who require it. The drugs should not be prescribed earlier in the treatment algorithm and patients receiving LABA should be regularly monitored by their clinician.

Anti IgE therapy

Xolair® (omalizumab) is a monclonal antibody directed against the IgE molecule. It is a new class of drug which is licensed in moderate to severe asthma in patients ages twelve and older. A blood test is done to see if a person has allergic asthma and to determine how high their blood IgE is. The drug licence states that IgE levels need to be within a certain range, patients whose levels are too high or too low ought not receive it. Xolair® is reserved for patients who are not controlled by high doses of inhaled steroids, daily oral steroids and other controller medication. Xolair® helps reduce the number of asthma attacks in people with asthma who still have poorly controlled symptoms, despite high doses of inhaled steroids. The FDA and European Medicines Agency approved Xolair® in June 2003. It is believed that the drug works by inhibiting the binding of IgE to the high-affinity IgE receptor (FcåRI) on the surface of mast cells and basophils. Reduction in surface-bound IgE on FcåRI-bearing cells limits the degree of release of mediators of the allergic response. Treatment with Xolair® also reduces the number of FcåRI receptors on basophils in atopic patients.

Xolair® comes as a subcutaneous injection. It should be administered in a doctor's clinic or hospital. Patients should read the medication guide before starting Xolair®, which is generally reserved for the most severely affected patients.

Side effects of Xolair® include:

- ✳ Anaphylaxis.
- ✳ Patients should not use Xolair® if they have had a previous allergic reaction to Xolair®, or if they are allergic to any of its ingredients.

* In clinical studies 0.5 percent of patients receiving Xolair® developed cancer, compared to 0.2 percent of patients receiving placebo.

* In patients less than 12 years of age, the most commonly observed side effects in asthma studies that had a less than 1 percent difference between Xolair® and placebo were joint pain (8 percent), general pain (7 percent), leg pain (4 percent), fatigue (3 percent), dizziness (3 percent), fracture (2 percent), arm pain (2 percent), itching (2 percent), inflammation of the skin (2 percent), and earache (2 percent).

* In asthma studies, the most common side effects in patients, who either needed to stop Xolair® or needed medical attention, were injection site reaction (45 percent), viral infections (23 percent), upper respiratory tract infection (20 percent), sinusitis (16 percent), headache (15 percent), and sore throat (11 percent). These side effects were seen at the same rates in Xolair®-treated patients as in patients in the control group who received placebo.

* Xolair® should not be thought of as a rescue medicine and should not be used to treat sudden asthma attacks. Xolair® is not a substitute for the medicines patients are already taking. Patients must not change or stop taking any of their other asthma medicines unless their doctor tells them to do so. Patients may not see an improvement in their asthma control for several weeks/months after beginning treatment.

In a recent study from Texas, of over 600 children with severe asthma, patients were randomised to receive either Xolair® (421) or placebo (206). Over the twenty-four week fixed-steroid phase, Xolair®, injected two to four times weekly, reduced the rate of clinically significant asthma exacerbations by 31 percent versus placebo. Over a period of fifty-two weeks, the exacerbation rate was significantly reduced by 43 percent versus placebo and oral or inhaled steroid doses were reduced. Xolair® significantly reduced severe exacerbations. Over a period of fifty-two weeks, Xolair® had an acceptable safety profile, with no difference in overall incidence of adverse events compared with placebo.

What is immunotherapy?

Immunotherapy is practised widely in Europe and in the US by allergists. However, immunotherapy had a bad start in Ireland and the UK in the 1950s, where it was associated with fatalities due to anaphylaxis. While other allergy treatments address only the symptoms of allergic disease, immunotherapy is the only available treatment that has the potential to modify the natural course of allergic disease. It has the potential to induce tolerance, where IgG antibodies are produced instead of the typical IgE. Typically, it requires a three to five-year individually tailored regimen of subcutaneous injections (SCIT) or sublingual treatments (SLIT), which may result in long-term benefits. Recent research suggests that patients who complete immunotherapy may continue to see benefits for years to come. Immunotherapy is not suitable for everybody or every allergic condition, and it may not be effective in those patients deemed suitable. However it offers allergy sufferers the chance to eventually reduce or stop symptomatic/rescue medication. The therapy is indicated for people who are extremely allergic or who cannot avoid specific allergens. For example, they may not be able to live a normal life and completely avoid pollen, dust mites, mould spores, pet dander, insect venom, and certain other common triggers of allergic reactions. Currently, immunotherapy is not indicated for food or medicinal allergies. However, in the near future it may become an option for those with specific food allergies, e.g. peanut. Immunotherapy is typically individually tailored and administered by an allergist. Injection schedules are available in some healthcare systems and can be prescribed by family physicians. This therapy is particularly useful for people with allergic rhinitis.

The therapy is likely to be successful if it begins early in life or soon after the allergy develops for the first time. Immunotherapy involves a series of injections (shots) given regularly for several years by an allergist in a hospital clinic. In the past, this was called a serum, but this is an incorrect name. Most allergists now call this mixture an allergy extract. The first shots contain very tiny amounts of the allergen or antigen to which you are allergic. With progressively increasing dosages over time, your body will adjust to the allergen and become less sensitive to it. This process is called desensitisation.

A recently approved sublingual tablet, Grazax®, containing a grass pollen extract, is similarly effective, with few side effects, and can be self-administered at home, including by those patients who also suffer from allergic asthma, a condition which precludes the use of injection-based desensitisation. Similar sublingual products are currently being investigated in clinical trials for dust allergic individuals who have allergic rhinitis and asthma. Oral desensitisation is being evaluated in research trials for peanut allergic children.

Can asthma cause lung damage?

The short answer is yes, but rarely. It is widely believed that persistent inflammation of the airways can cause structural changes leading to fixed narrowing of the bronchial tubes. The process is known as airway remodelling. This will be apparent on a pulmonary function test which will show an obstructive pattern without a bronchodilator response. Experts believe that inadequate control of asthma may lead to this fixed obstruction in some patients. Also, bronchial hyper-responsiveness may persist while symptoms abate.

If asthma is not controlled, individuals may suffer from recurrent chest infections. Sometimes, an infection becomes chronic and can lead to another form of airway damage called bronchiectasis. This is characterised by irreversible dilation of the airway, poor clearance of mucus and susceptibility in that area to further bouts of infection. In uncomplicated asthma the cough is typically episodic and dry, whereas in bronchiectasis the cough is persistent and moist. In bronchiectasis a chest X-ray may be normal, and the condition is best diagnosed using Chest CT (salami slice x-ray images through the lung). In a study published in 2010, we found that in Ireland approximately 2.6 children per 100,000 have this condition. Asthma and bronchiectasis co-existed in the same patient in nearly 20 percent of cases.

In normal childhood and adolescence our lung capacity increases as we grow until we reach adulthood when height and body growth ceases. In middle age there is a natural decline in lung function which continues into old age. This phenomena generally goes unnoticed. However, if there is an underlying chest problem then the process of decline in lung function may be exaggerated or occur prematurely. Chronic obstructive pulmonary disease (COPD) or chronic bronchitis/emphysema is a condition that predominantly affects middle-aged and older people who have smoked cigarettes. The symptoms can be quite similar to asthma and there can be an overlap between the two common conditions. There is now an emerging body of evidence which supports the theory that although environmental exposures are important, the roots of this condition lie in antenatal conditions and nutrition in the first year of life.

Together with smoking, the lung function attained in early adulthood seems to be one of the strongest predictors of chronic obstructive pulmonary disease. In order to investigate whether lung function in early adulthood is, in turn, affected by airway function measured shortly after birth, 1,200 infants were enrolled at birth in the Tucson Children's Respiratory Study between 1980 and 1984. Specialised infant pulmonary function tests were performed at three months. Standard measurements of lung function were performed in these participants at ages eleven, sixteen and twenty-two years. They found that participants who had low levels of infant lung function had lower values as adults. The magnitude and significance of this effect did not change after additional adjustment for wheeze, smoking, atopy or parental asthma. They concluded that poor airway function shortly after birth should be recognised as a risk factor for airflow obstruction in young adults and postulated that prevention of COPD might need to start in foetal life.

Another recent study from Australia also provided epidemiological evidence to suggest that events in childhood that influence lung growth constitute a significant risk for COPD. Subjects of the Melbourne Asthma Study were recruited at the age of seven from a 1957 birth cohort and were assessed regularly until the age of fifty. At recruitment, subjects were classified as having no history of wheeze, intermittent asthma (such as viral-induced wheezing), persistent asthma (in the absence of illness), or severe asthma. Of the surviving members of the original group, 197 answered a detailed questionnaire and underwent lung function testing for the current study. Subjects who were classified as having severe asthma in childhood had a much higher statistical risk of developing COPD (32 times that of children without asthma). Interestingly, children with mild asthma were not at increased risk of developing adult obstructive lung disease. Children with more severe asthma features tend to have predisposing risk factors (like atopy) and continue to have symptoms of wheeze well into adult life. Lung function in children with severe asthma is reduced in childhood years and declined at a normal rate in adult life to levels consistent with adult obstructive lung disease. The authors concluded that in severe asthma where lung function is initially reduced, it gradually deteriorates to levels consistent with a diagnosis of COPD. The CAMP cohort study has also provided insights into lung function attained by childhood asthmatics during adulthood. Worryingly, only 20 percent of those who reached adulthood had normal lung function, 25 percent exhibited diminished lung function, 24 percent had initially normal lung function but entered an early decline, and 28 percent had initially abnormal lung function and experienced an early decline. The authors concluded that those exhibiting early decline in lung function may represent the evolution of patients from asthma to COPD.

> **Will my child outgrow their asthma?**

In the past, children's asthma tended to be considered a trivial disorder because it was mistakenly assumed that most sufferers outgrew their condition by the teenage years. This has been proven to be a myth and while many children's asthma improves with age, there is no guarantee that your child will outgrow their asthma. In fact, most adults with asthma had symptoms in childhood. The course of asthma in a given individual may be extremely variable over childhood and may go through periods of relapse and remission. For example, parents may notice that their child's asthma symptoms disappear over the summer months only to return again in autumn. By adolescence, a significant proportion of people find that their symptoms have disappeared; however, their asthma may recur in their thirties and forties. In general, studies have consistently found that boys have a better chance of outgrowing asthma than girls. The older the child is when symptoms begin, the less chance they have to outgrow the condition. Females are at higher risk of having persisting asthma. The presence of concurrent allergic conditions, e.g. rhinitis and eczema, and wheezy episodes outside of viral illnesses also increases the risk.

It was thought that approximately two-thirds of children outgrow their asthma. However, this prognosis may not be so favourable. The Childhood Asthma Management Programme, a cohort study of over 1,000 children with asthma who have been followed from the early 1990's, many of whom are young adults now. Their clinical course and lung function have been monitored regularly over the course of the study. Of the original cohort 463 had reached the age of 21 years. Surprisingly, only 12 percent had remitted by then, 30 percent complained of periodic symptoms and 58 percent had persistent symptoms. In those with residual asthma, 50 percent were on controller medications and 90 percent used relievers. Risks for severe asthma included older age of symptom onset, sensitisation to indoor allergens and diminished lung function.

Can hormones influence asthma?

Some children with asthma may appear small and physically immature in the early teenage years. Naturally, parents will be concerned that asthma therapy may be somehow related to this. Generally speaking, this phenomenon is unrelated to treatment. It has been documented that children with asthma have delayed skeletal maturity and tend to enter puberty later than their non-asthmatic peers. For example, at thirteen years, males may not show any signs of puberty and have the skeletal age of an eleven-year-old. In essence it means they have two years of additional growing to do. Ultimately, all asthmatic children will grow to a normal adult height.

Some teenage girls with asthma may find that, in the days before their period, their asthma control deteriorates. This phenomenon is known as pre-menstrual asthma. The mechanisms that lay behind this remain unclear: female hormones such as oestrogen clearly play a role, but oestrogen itself is not the culprit in triggering the symptoms of asthma. Rather, it's the variation of oestrogen from high to low levels that may cause an increase in inflammation of the airways. In the days before a period, oestrogen levels drop and it is believed that this fall increases susceptibility to the individual's specific triggers. This type of asthma is diagnosed by peak flow monitoring over several months and detecting a reproducible drop or increased fluctuation of readings in the days leading up to the onset of a period. Sometimes in severe cases, oestrogen treatment in the form of the pill may be required. The physiologic effect of female hormones may in part explain the gender switch that occurs in asthma from where more males have asthma in childhood and more females have asthma as adults.

What do I do during an asthma attack?

Follow the Asthma Society of Ireland's 'Five Minute Rule': if your child becomes suddenly wheezy and breathless, give them their reliever inhaler immediately.

Then:

a) Don't panic! Stay calm and reassure your child.

b) Get your child to sit on a comfortable chair and loosen any tight clothing.

c) Do not cuddle or put your arms around them.

d) Encourage slow and calm breathing.

If there is no immediate improvement, give the reliever inhaler (two puffs of an MDI or one puff of a dry powder inhaler) every minute for five minutes.

If there is no improvement, call your doctor, GP out-of-hours service, or local Children's Emergency Department, or dial 999.

Continue to give reliever medication until you start to receive medical attention. If you already have a written asthma management plan and have been given a back-up prescription for oral steroids, take a dose as directed and continue to use your reliever medication.

Seek medical attention if you have any doubts about your child's condition. Don't forget to bring your child's current inhalers and any other medications that they are taking. Remember that an asthma attack reflects a failure in asthma control and that you will need to make an appointment with your GP or asthma clinic to review triggers, inhaler technique and medication.

What are asthma clinics?

Asthma clinics are set up specifically to manage asthma. They can be based in your GP's surgery, consultant clinic or in hospital. They comprise a number of healthcare professionals who have specific expertise in the diagnosis and management of asthma. A typical asthma clinic will consist of a doctor and nurse. In hospitals or consultant clinics there will often be a pulmonary function technician, who will perform spirometry and allergy tests. These tests may be performed by an asthma nurse in a general practice setting. The key component of an asthma clinic is expertise; a good asthma clinic should be treating many patients with the condition, not just an occasional case. The team members will be proficient in treating asthma, be familiar with the latest treatment guidelines and be capable of educating the child or their parent. The patient will be provided with written or web-based educational material at diagnosis, they will have been prescribed the appropriate inhaler device and medication and a date for follow-up. The patient ought to receive a written treatment plan and depending on their age will be given a peak-flow meter.

What is a peak flow meter?

A peak flow meter is a simple device that can be used at home by a school-aged child. It is a small, hand-held device used to monitor a person's ability to breathe out air. It measures the airflow through the bronchi and thus the degree of obstruction in the airways. The technique is relatively simple and involves a forced exhalation into the device following a deep inspiration. Your child's peak flow is determined by their ethnicity, gender, age and height. The best of three readings are taken morning and evening. The results are often plotted on a graph or on a computer spreadsheet. An individual's personal best reading is determined by taking multiple readings over time whilst the asthma is under good control. The peak low traffic light system will usually run as follows: Green (PEF between 80 and 100 percent of personal best), Yellow (PEF between 60 and 80 percent of personal best), orange (PEF between 40 and 60 percent of personal best) and red (less than 40 percent of personal best). Your child's personal best peak flow will increase as they get older and taller. In an asthma attack the PEF will drop dramatically and may improve with a reliever. I don't routinely recommend a PEF meter for milder asthmatics because I have found that, over time, as their asthma becomes well controlled they stop taking routine readings. I find a peak flow meter particularly useful for patients with more difficult asthma, particularly those who don't perceive their symptoms very well and who tend to experience sudden attacks. The PEF in this scenario can provide an early warning system where treatment can be intensified in advance of the development of an asthma attack in the hope of aborting it. I also use a PEF meter to help me determine whether symptoms are due to asthma or whether in fact a patient has asthma at all.

How do I use a peak flow meter?

Readings are best taken in the standing position and prior to the administration of any asthma medication. Set the cursor to zero. Inhale deeply then place your mouth tightly around the mouth piece and blow out fast and hard (I often ask children to pretend that they are blowing out candles on a birthday cake). Note the first reading, set the cursor at zero again and repeat the procedure. The best of three readings is taken. It is important to ensure that your child makes a consistently good effort each time. There is a natural variation in peak flow readings between morning and evening. Research has shown that airway calibre is widest at 4PM and narrowest at 4AM In asthma, this difference is exaggerated. Instead of varying by about 10 percent, the airway width can vary by 20 percent or more. This is a sign that asthma is active and unstable, and that the airways are twitchy and irritable.

What is a written treatment plan?

Most guidelines recommend a written asthma plan so that the patient or their parents have a record of the main treatment recommendations following their consultation with their doctor or asthma nurse. It will outline the type, dose and frequency of preventative treatment as well as the way to use reliever medication. Often a traffic light system is used where peak flow and symptoms are used to help the patient manage their own asthma and determine what level of treatment is required.

Although a written action plan is recommended for children, up until recently its independent value was questionable. A study published in 2010 examined whether providing a written action plan coupled with a prescription improved adherence to medications and other recommendations. two hundred and nineteen children who presented with acute asthma symptoms received either a standard prescription or written action plan. The main outcome was adherence to preventative treatment over twenty eight days. Other outcomes included requirement of oral corticosteroids, salbutamol use, medical follow-up, emergency room visits and assessment of control. The authors concluded that the provision of a written action plan significantly increased patient adherence to inhaled and oral corticosteroids and asthma control, as well as physicians' recommendations for controller medication and medical follow-up, thus supporting its independent value.

Asthma at school

When your child starts in primary school it is very important that their principal and class teacher know about their condition. Because asthma prevalence is so high in Ireland, your child will not be unique and there will be many other children at school who also have the condition. The class teacher must be informed of the potential triggers that may exist at school and what to do if your child develops symptoms suddenly. It can be a good idea to give them a copy of your written asthma treatment plan. There is no need for preventative/controller treatment to be taken at school as they will normally be taken morning and evening before and after the school day. Unfortunately, schools in Ireland differ quite considerably in terms of their attitude to asthma and the administration of reliever medications. A hundred and fifty school principals participated in a study conducted by the Asthma Society of Ireland. The study found that 85 percent of schools had children with asthma attending, and 81 percent had no specific guidelines for asthma. A quarter of schools interviewed had dealt with an asthma attack. Only one-third of schools said that they talked to parents of children with asthma on an annual basis.

However, the Asthma Society of Ireland has an excellent booklet which can form the basis of any discussion you have with the school authorities. Older primary and secondary school children ought to be allowed carry their own reliever medications and should be allowed to take their reliever before planned exercise and when symptoms dictate.

It is also important for children to have an asthma check-up prior to going back to school, because this virtually always heralds the start of the respiratory virus season for that winter. Adherence with preventative/controller and inhaler technique should be assessed. As children get older the type of inhaler device may need to change.

Asthma and holidays

People often worry that asthma flare-ups may occur whilst away from home and are not sure whether it is safe to go on holiday. Prior planning is important, especially when travelling abroad. Air travel is generally not a problem. However, if your child's asthma is not properly controlled, air conditioning can irritate the lungs. During mid-term breaks and summer holidays flights are frequently full with many children aboard. It is an ideal environment for the spread of viral infections, and it is not unusual for children to become ill at the start of a holiday as the result of viral infections contracted on the flight. It is generally a good idea to investigate the potential environmental triggers that may prevail at the location under consideration. It would be wise to avoid locations that are heavily polluted or where there can be high pollen counts if these have been issues for your child previously. One also has to be careful when renting holiday homes because damp or mouldy conditions or dusty environments can all exacerbate asthma.

A check-up with your doctor or asthma nurse provides an opportunity to have your control assessed, treatment reviewed and an outline of your written management plan explained. Your asthma ought to be under good control and it is generally not a good idea to step down treatment prior to a holiday. A letter from your physician detailing the diagnosis and treatment may be useful in advising local physicians in the event of an attack. Sometimes your doctor may prescribe a back-up script for a short course of oral steroids. If you have a nebuliser that operates from the mains, you need to make sure that the A/C current at your holiday destination is compatible. Bring the appropriate adaptors and current transformers.

When travelling, ensure that you carry your medications in your hand luggage. Make sure that your inhalers are in date and that you have sufficient medication for the holiday. If travelling abroad, make sure that your holiday insurance covers asthma and if travelling in Europe, be sure to apply for your European Health Insurance Card. If your child has allergies please take the appropriate precautions. Children with a peanut allergy should take the following steps to stay safe on an airplane: check whether nuts are served as a snack; if so notify your carrier; bring your own food for the flight and ensure that you have access to your adrenalin and antihistamine when you are travelling; wipe down your table, head rest and arm rest.

> **Asthma and exercise**

Exertional symptoms may be a manifestation of poor asthma control or may occur in isolation, a condition known as 'exercise-induced asthma'. Symptoms such as dry cough, chest tightness/pain, excessive breathlessness and wheeze can develop shortly after exertion. Children may complain of not being able to keep up with peers in games and sports. Some may say they don't like games or avoid participating; others may opt to play in less active positions in team sports, e.g. goalkeeper. These symptoms can lead to problems with socialisation or self-esteem in some children. It is important that your child's PE teacher or sports coach is aware of their condition and medications.

Typically these symptoms are worse with track and field sports such as athletics, GAA, rugby, hockey and soccer. This is thought to be due to the effects of fast breathing of cold, damp or very dry air mainly through the mouth and the relative lack of the warming and humidification effect generated by nose breathing which normally occurs at rest. For many years swimming was recommended as an exercise for people with asthma. The rationale was that the air was warm and humid in an indoor pool and thus was less irritating to the lung. Many asthmatics find swimming an excellent way to maintain fitness without suffering any ill effects from chlorine. Despite the theories linking the development of asthma to chlorinated swimming pools, swimming is still recommended as an exercise option for asthmatics. If chlorine causes irritation of the airways, try swimming in an non-chlorinated pool e.g. ozone or even sea swimming. Where exercise symptoms reflect overall poor control of asthma, it will be necessary to review an individual's controller treatment, inhaler technique and adherence to treatment. Isolated exercise related asthma can be improved or prevented by the following:

a) A warm-up session before the match or training.
b) Wearing a scarf around nose and mouth in cold air, where possible.
c) Administration of a short-acting bronchodilator taken fifteen minutes prior to planned exertion.

For more resistant forms of the condition, inhaled steroids, anti-leukoriene drugs and long-acting bronchodilators may be useful. Children with asthma should be able to fully participate in sport without experiencing symptoms. Many elite sportspeople have asthma and surveys of Olympians have found a higher proportion of asthma than would be expected in the normal population.

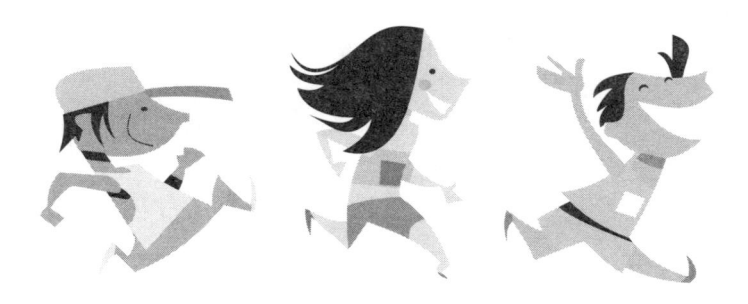

> **Does having asthma mean that my child can't participate in competitive sports?**

Many children and teenagers with asthma compete in sport at quite a high level. Indeed, asthma appears to be quite common in elite athletes. According to one study, at least one in six athletes representing the United States in the 1996 Olympic Games had a history of asthma, in contrast to the 5 percent prevalence given for the general population. Olympians have been shown to have consistently higher prevalence rates of asthma.

Out of 699 athletes, 117 (16.7 percent) were found to have a history of asthma, or to have used asthma medications, or both. seventy three (10.4 percent) of the athletes had active asthma, based on their need for asthma medication at the time of the games, or their need for medication on a permanent or semi-permanent basis. Among the Olympic athletes, asthma was most common among cyclists and mountain bikers and least common in athletes competing in badminton, beach volleyball, table tennis and volleyball. Interestingly, nearly 30 percent of the 1996 US Olympians who had asthma or took asthma medications won team or individual medals in their Olympic competition, faring as well as athletes without asthma (28.7 percent) who earned team or individual medals.

We all know that exercise is beneficial to both physical health and emotional wellbeing. Even if a child is not striving to be an Olympic athlete, it is expected that, with help of medication, all children with exercise-induced asthma should be able to exercise to their full ability.

> **Are asthma drugs prohibited by sports authorities?**

Certain drugs used for asthma have the potential to be anabolic (promote muscle gain). It may come as some surprise that it is the beta-agonist class, not inhaled steroids, that have been implicated. The World Anti-Doping Agency (WADA) has banned most forms of inhaled or oral beta agonists (these include formoterol, terbutaline, clenbuterol and acebuterol).

This includes those combined with an inhaled steroid in a single inhaler. Salbutamol by inhalation is permitted up to a ceiling dose of 1600 mcg per day (two puffs eight times daily), so too is Seretide (salmeterol + fluticazone in combination), however certification by a treating physician is required.

Oral salbutamol is banned. Certain other beta-adrenergicagonists (e.g. ephedrine, bitolterol, metaproterenol) are banned. Care must be taken with over the counter cold and flu remedies as they too can contain banned substances (pseudoephedrine). Caution must also be exercised using herbal preparations bought in food stores (e.g. Ma Huang), which contain stimulants useful for asthma but are banned.

Any child or young adult who participates in an amateur athletic event where drug testing may occur should check with their coach and physician regarding the status of any substance being used during competition.

> **Are ibuprofen and paracetamol safe for children with asthma?**

Aspirin-sensitive asthma is a rare type of asthma where asthma attacks are provoked by aspirin and other NSAIDs like ibuprofen and diclofenac. It mainly affects adults. It is commonly seen in females who also suffer from allergic rhinitis and may have nasal polyps. Symptoms consist of cough, wheeze, urticaria and swelling of the lips and face. Occasionally it can progress to full anaphylaxis. The antileukotriene drugs appear to be particularly beneficial for this condition. These days aspirin is virtually never prescribed for children because of a serious but rare side effect called Reye's Syndrome. However, other NSAIDs are used, particularly ibuprofen. It is available over the counter and is given to infants and children with fever or as a painkiller. Doctors are frequently asked whether it is safe to give ibuprofen to children with asthma. The answer is yes, most asthmatic children will not have any problem taking ibuprofen. In a recent systematic review of the relevant medical literature it was found that there exists a low risk for asthma-related morbidity associated with ibuprofen use in children and a possible protective and therapeutic effect compared with paracetamol. The study also found that acetaminophen use in children is associated with an increased risk for wheezing.

Subsequent studies specifically addressed the link between exposure to paracetamol during intrauterine life, childhood, and adult life and the risk of developing asthma. Children aged six to seven years from Phase Three of the International Study of Asthma and Allergies in Childhood programme were studied. Parents/guardians completed written questionnaires about symptoms of asthma, rhinoconjunctivitis and eczema, as well as several risk factors, including the use of paracetamol for fever in the child's first year of life and the frequency of paracetamol use in the past twelve months. In total 205,487 children from 73 centres in 31 countries were included in the study.

In the analysis, use of paracetamol for fever in the first year of life was associated with an increased risk of asthma symptoms when aged six to seven years. Current use of paracetamol was associated with a dose-dependent increased risk of asthma symptoms. Use of paracetamol was similarly associated with the risk of severe asthma symptoms. The authors concluded that paracetamol use, both in the first year of life and in children aged six to seven years, was also associated with an increased risk of symptoms of rhinoconjunctivitis and eczema. Critics argued that children with asthma get more respiratory infections and that paracetemol use is simply a reflection of that.

These findings led to further research. In 2010, a smaller study of 620 Australian children followed analphylaxis to determine if use of paracetamol in early life is an independent risk factor for childhood asthma. This birth cohort were followed until age seven. The researchers found that paracetamol had been used in 51 percent of children by twelve weeks of age and in 97 percent by two years. Between six and seven years, 80 percent were followed up; 30 percent had current asthma. Paracetamol use for non-respiratory causes was not associated with asthma. They concluded that even in children with a family history of allergic disease, no association could be found between early paracetamol use and risk of subsequent allergic disease and that there was no reason not give paracetamol to children with asthma who require pain relief or anti-fever medication.

> **Are there any new drugs being developed to treat asthma?**

Most asthma will still be successfully managed by standard methods including allergen and trigger avoidance, bronchodilators and inhaled steroids. New therapeutic strategies are emerging that may be beneficial to those with more severe forms of the disease. These will focus on particular key targets of the inflammatory response. These type of therapies have progressed more in the specialty of rheumatology and are known as 'the biologics'. They typically target antibodies, cytokines or their receptors. In asthma, the most successful biologic is the monoclonal IgG antibody directed against IgE (Xolair®), which blocks IgE binding to the high affinity receptor for IgE (Fc R1) on mast cells and basophils. It prevents the binding of natural specific IgE to its receptor. Thus when an allergen is encountered, the mast cells does not destabilise or release its inflammatory contents. This has passed through clinical trials, FDA and EMA regulatory processes and is clinically available now. It has become the therapy of choice for suitable patients with severe asthma. A vaccine therapy is under development, which is designed to raise protective antibodies against IgE. The immunotherapeutic agent RP102 is undergoing safety trials in humans.

Other biologics under development for asthma include an anti-IL-5 antibody, which opposes the action of eosinophils, cells that are pivotal effectors of allergic airway inflammation. In a clincical trial the anti IL-5 antibody (mepolizumab) caused significant decreases in airway eosinophils but this did not translate into improved clinical outcomes. Further back along the inflammatory pathway, efforts address IL-4 a cytokine produced by the Th2 class of lymphocytes that result in the proliferation of clones of cells that produce IgE. Blocking the effects of IL-4 can be achieved by complexing it to its receptor. IL-4 receptors have been safely administered to human asthmatics and in two small studies produced a net decrease in the doses of inhaled steroid required to control patients' asthma. However, in larger scale studies, the agent failed to influence the primary endpoint which was lung function. Other targets being evaluated are vaccines directed against IL-4, and antibodies directed against IL-9, IL-10 and IL-12. In some subtypes of asthma, the key effector cell is the neutrophil, whose behaviour is governed by a completely different set of cytokines. Tumour necrosis factor alpha (TNF) is an important regulator of neutrophil activity. Agents have been developed which can block its action and clinical trials have yielded mixed results in this form of asthma.

Interferons are important regulators of Th1 mediated immune responses. Trials with subcutaneous interferon gamma (IFN) in asthmatics have been disappointing. However, there are other interferons which seem more promising. Small clinical trials with IFN and IFN when given subcutaneously by injection over eighteen months were shown to be effective in the treatment of severe oral steroid-dependent asthma. In one study the investigators demonstrated a switch back to a Th1 cytokine profile in the blood of recipients.

Mast cells have been targets for therapy in asthma for many years. The mast cell stabilisers sodium dicromoglycate and nedocromil have been available for many years. New, more specific targets on mast cells include CD63, which regulates signalling within the cell, antibodies to CD63 have been shown to inhibit FCR1 mediated mast cell activation. There are certain enzymes which are involved in mast cell activation called SRC tyrosine kinases. Compounds have been developed which interfere with their function and prevent mast cell activation in the presence of an allergen. In clinical trials, the compound R112 reduced inflammatory nasal responses in patients with seasonal allergic rhinitis exposed to a high pollen count.

Finally, I believe that advances in genetics will permit the prediction of responses to particular therapies e.g. bronchodilators, inhaled steroids and antileukotriene drugs using gene-chip technology. New non-invasive biomarkers such as exhaled NO will be developed that will also identify patient subtypes who will benefit from specific interventions.

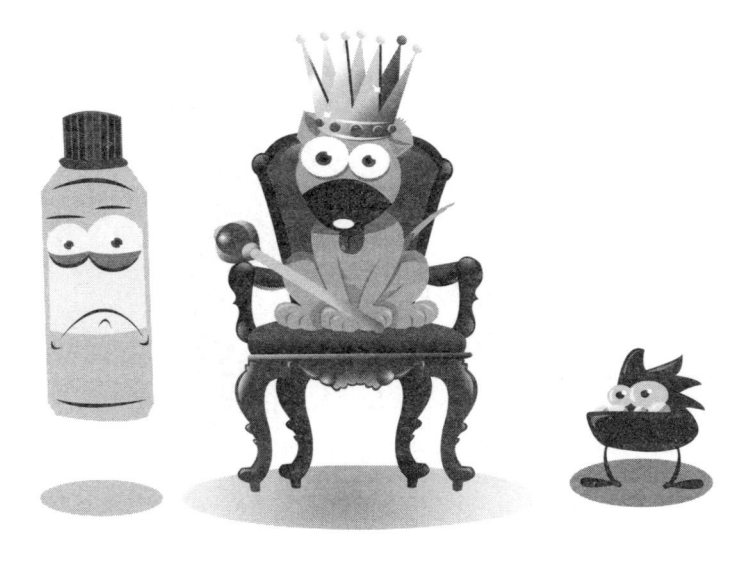

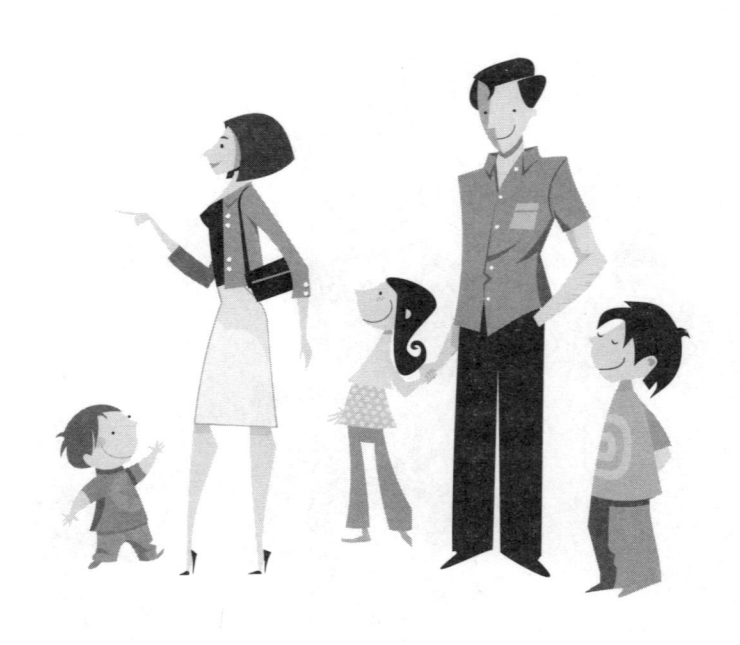

Clinical Scenarios from the Asthma Society Helpline

ASTHMA SOCIETY OF IRELAND
1850 44 54 64

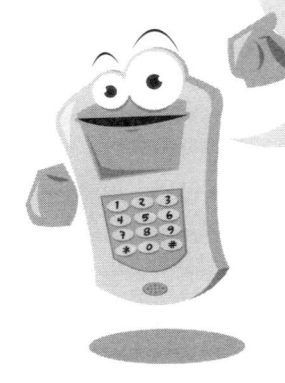

Q: I called the Asthma Society Helpline because I am really concerned for my little girl, who is eight years old and has had asthma since infancy. She has been well all summer but I'm dreading her going back to school because she gets sick every year in September. I wanted to know if there is anything I can do to help her stay well when she goes back to school?

A: The asthma nurse I spoke to really understood my concerns and explained to me that it is very common for children's asthma to worsen in September. There are many reasons for this, including exposure to new allergens and triggers such as colds and viruses. But also other things like children's excitement at being back in school and back with friends and maybe having to manage their own medication or having to rely on a teacher rather than a parent to take charge of inhalers. The nurse asked me in detail about Aoife's medication and I told her that Aoife takes a brown inhaler all the time and is really very well on that. She sometimes needs a blue inhaler but that's rare.

She explained to me that there are a number of steps I can take to help my daughter continue to have good control of her asthma. It is important to have Aoife's asthma reviewed by her doctor prior to school commencement, as during the winter months colds and flu cause a winter-time threat to children with asthma, and ask for a written personal action plan. The plan should include information that I need in order to keep control of Aoife's asthma including: details on her medications and the importance of taking her medication on a daily basis; how to tell when her symptoms are getting worse; what I can do about it and most especially, what to do during an attack. She told me I should ask my GP's practice nurse to check Aoife's inhaler technique. The nurse suggested that it would be a good idea for me to visit Aoife's school and make sure her teacher is aware that Aoife has asthma and that going back to school in itself is a trigger for Aoife, as is playing outdoors in the cold. I should also ask if there is a school policy on asthma in place, or what measures are in place if a child has an asthma attack.

The nurse also advised that I use an Asthma Society of Ireland school card to record essential details that the school needs to know about Aoife's health and treatment. She said that it is imperative for Aoife to carry her blue reliever at all times, and that a blue reliever is left in school and labelled clearly with her name. The nurse suggested that the school should contact the Asthma Society of Ireland for a copy of their booklet, 'Best Practice Asthma Management Guidelines for Primary Schools in Ireland'. And finally, I was advised to keep Aoife at home if she is not well enough to attend. Altogether I feel much more confident now that school is about to start and I have an appointment to speak to Aoife's teacher.

> **Q:** My six-year-old son has asthma and allergic rhinitis. He has been very well controlled for the past two years and managed to reduce his medications and he is now old enough to take his inhaler directly without a spacer. However, he became very unwell about three weeks ago and I have increased his medications to what he was originally prescribed. He is still no better. What should I do?

A: I rang the Asthma Helpline and explained the situation. The nurse asked me what symptoms he was experiencing. I explained to her he coughs a lot and gets very short of breath. He wakes at night coughing and his nose is dripping constantly. He is using his blue reliever more often and is getting less relief from it. The nurse said that my son's asthma was out of control. I told her how Mark has never had an actual attack but that when his asthma goes out of control, he becomes worn out and generally unwell. He can't lie flat and his sleep is disrupted, he has no appetite and becomes quite irritable. The asthma nurse said what I was describing was an acute exacerbation of asthma and said that I should bring my son to my GP as soon as possible and address a number of issues such as:

1. That I have been changing his medications (increasing and decreasing the doses depending on how well Mark has been) without a formal asthma management plan.

2. His nasal allergy needs to be addressed either with a nasal spray or an antihistamine.

3. That he needs to have his inhaler technique checked and to start using his spacer again as it is unlikely that he is receiving sufficient drug to his airways using the inhaler alone.

I had used a peak flow meter and diary before with Mark and the asthma nurse suggested that I start using them again, as this will take the guesswork out of knowing how well my son is. She said she would send me a new diary. She also suggested that I replace the chamber device as my previous one was two years old, and explained how this would not only improve the efficiency of the medication but reduce the side effects in the mouth. I had noticed that Mark has had dreadful thrush in his mouth since stopping using the chamber. She stressed the importance of adherence with his medication plan, recognising the signs and symptoms of deteriorating asthma and when to get help.

She also said that even when a child is well, it is recommended that they undergo routine asthma reviews every six months. Mark has not been seen by a doctor in two years! The asthma nurse advised me to make an appointment with my GP to review Mark's asthma. She suggested that at this next visit I should ask about a personalised written asthma plan for Mark, a review of medication both for his chest and nose, and a follow-up appointment to assess how well this plan is working.

I felt a lot better having spoken to the asthma nurse and realised that, although I have been managing my son's asthma reasonably well for a number of years, there are more structured ways of doing so. I have made an appointment to visit my GP with the intention of implementing the asthma nurse's suggestions.

> **Q:** I have started a new job as a child minder. I now care for an eighteen-month-old girl in my home, Monday to Friday. My husband smokes. We have a cat and a rabbit which stay indoors. I am now worried as the child has been chesty on a number of occasions since September, which coincides with her coming to us. Have I caused this child to have asthma?

A: A diagnosis of asthma can be difficult to obtain in children under the age of two. At least one child in five will have 'wheezing' during their early years but do not necessarily go on to develop asthma. The diagnosis is usually made on a pattern of symptoms over a period of time. It will be based on a family history, the pattern of symptoms, a physical examination of the chest, and in older children a breathing test and a trial of treatment. A number of triggers can cause wheezing and coughing in this age group, particularly infection with respiratory viruses.

Different children react to different triggers, which parents or carers can gradually recognise and it would be beneficial to eliminate avoidable triggers. Passive smoking causes health problems for everyone, therefore it might be appropriate to confine smoking to one area in your house where you and the child won't go. Even better would be to urge your husband to smoke outdoors and maintain a smoke-free house. Stopping smoking of course, would be the best advice! If your husband was willing to be persuaded, his GP can offer assistance in the form of nicotine replacement therapy or other therapies or strategies to help quit. Alternatively, one can contact the National Smokers Quitline on 1850 201 203.

Some children with asthma are allergic to furry animals and occasionally birds. It might be best to keep the pets out of the area where you will be caring for the child. Frequent washing of the pets is also recommended. I would suggest you take the appropriate measures as outlined above and have a discussion with the child's mother expressing your concerns.

> **Q:** I am a primary school teacher and a child with an allergy to peanuts has just joined my class. She carries an Anapen. Would you please outline how to use it in the case of an emergency?

A: Anapens are primarily for self-use by the person who is at risk of a reaction. Be familiar with the guidelines of allergy set down by your school. Adrenalin is used for severe allergic reactions where there are breathing problems, significant swelling of the tongue which may compromise the airway, or where the child becomes unconscious because of low blood pressure (shock).

Instructions for use:

1. Remove the black needle cap.
2. Remove the black safety cap from the red firing button.
3. Hold the Anapen against the upper outer aspect of the thigh and press the red firing button (it is better to inject directly onto skin).
4. Hold the Anapen in position for ten seconds (this allows the full dose of adrenalin to be injected).

5 Remove and dispose of the Anapen safely (do not try to retract needle).

6 Gently massage the injection site.

7 Medical help should be sought as soon as possible, as relapse can occur within a few hours and/or further management may be required.

A repeat injection may be given after five minutes if the effects of acute allergic reaction have not started to settle.

Q: My doctor has diagnosed me with asthma. How can he be sure? He did no tests.

A: Though there is no straightforward definition of asthma and no tests that can diagnose asthma with absolute certainty, the average uncomplicated case of asthma is fairly easy to diagnose in adults and children over the age of five years.

Much of the diagnosis depends on what doctors call 'taking a good history'. This means asking you about the actual symptoms and their triggers, and when you first noticed them. It is important to give an accurate account and it may be useful to write down your symptoms before you go to the doctor.

A thorough medical history and examination may be followed by a number of essential tests, such as lung function tests with reversibility and allergy tests. Also, you may be given a peak flow monitor and diary asked to check your own peak flow at home every morning and evening for three to four weeks. The pattern of results and your response to treatment may help in deciding whether you have asthma or not.

Q: My child's vaccinations are due. How safe are they?

A: Vaccinations are safe and have been used for many years by millions of people around the world, with very few side effects. All children should be vaccinated in accordance with the National Immunisation Guidelines for Ireland. There are very few children who cannot receive their routine vaccines. Children with asthma are more at risk of coughs, colds and viral infections. Viral infections are the commonest reason for worsening asthma in children and the commonest reason for hospital admissions. Flu is a seasonal viral infection, hence the importance of influenza vaccination each October.

Q: We have just moved into a rented apartment and within a few days I noticed my little girl's allergies have become worse. She now complains of tightness of chest and a stuffed nose. Do you know of a place where I can buy products, like a powder or a spray, that kill dust mites?

A: Before anybody could recommend any products, it would be best to examine why your child has experienced a worsening of their allergies. One of the reasons may be the condition of the apartment that you have moved into. For example, is it very dusty? Are there carpets? Were any pets there prior to you moving? How is it heated? These questions should be addressed before any treatment is recommended. I would suggest that you keep a diary of your child's symptoms and when they are occurring. Monitoring her peak flow morning and night will also help with the managing of her asthma. With this in mind, go and visit your GP and let him know of her deterioration. After taking an accurate history and measuring her lung function, an allergy test – either a skin or blood test to identify potential triggers – may be requested to help your GP decide on how best to manage her asthma and nasal allergy. Inhaled treatment for her nose and lungs may also be prescribed and it is imperative that you are shown how to take them and told how important adherence to treatment is. It is also recommended that you are given a follow-up appointment to review her progress. A written management plan ought to be in place to help you to manage your child's condition.

> **Q:** My son was in hospital recently with asthma and received nebulised therapy. It worked very well for him so I now want to get a nebuliser. Where will I get it and what medicine do I put in it? How often can I use it?

A: Inhaler devices are the first preference for use in the control of asthma. Nebulised treatments deliver large amounts of medicine in vapour via a mask or mouthpiece. It is driven by compressed air or oxygen. Nebulised treatment may be prescribed in the acute situation in the emergency department. It may also be prescribed as part of maintenance therapy by your GP or hospital consultant. If prescribed in the acute situation, the need for nebulised therapy recedes as the exacerbation diminishes. Recent studies have shown that one can achieve equivalent drug delivery to the airways with a large volume spacer. Indeed, most children's emergency departments, have now replaced nebulisers with spacing devices like the Volumatic® through which they administer high doses of inhaled Salbutamol.

Q: I have a strong suspicion that my son, who is fifteen years old and has asthma, has started to smoke. What should I do?

A: If it is only a suspicion then I suggest you do not confront your son as he may become defensive and you may damage your relationship with him. If you have seen the evidence then tell him you know he is smoking; let him know of your concerns, especially because of his asthma. Restrict your conversation to your concerns for his health and how you feel about it, but avoid making judgements or forecasts about him. Let him know about programmes and methods that are available to help smokers stop. He will have to make the decision to stop himself, and nagging him may not be helpful. Smoking is highly addictive which is why it is difficult to stop, and most smokers start in their teenage years. So being supportive and encouraging is the only way you can help your son. Keep the relationship between you friendly and open, regardless of the outcome.

Q: My doctor has prescribed my fourteen-month-old daughter a blue inhaler and a spacer with a face mask. He thinks she may have asthma. She gets so upset and cries when I give it to her. Have you any advice?

A: It can be really difficult to persuade young children to take medication via a spacer and face mask. However, with a lot of patience, positive reinforcement and distraction techniques, it will get easier. I would suggest that you start slowly by introducing your child to the spacer and mask again:

- ✳ Leave it visible and within easy reach so that the spacer and facemask is not something to be feared when suddenly it appears.
- ✳ Decorate it with stickers to make it more appealing.
- ✳ Let your child put it on her favourite teddy or doll's face.
- ✳ Slowly build up her tolerance of having the mask near her face, on her face and eventually covering her nose and mouth.
- ✳ Obviously this works better if practiced when she does not need medication rather than waiting until medication is needed.

Children of this age respond to distraction techniques, for example singing songs, reading books and playing counting games. Counting games work very well for slightly older children, counting out loud to your daughter as your daughter takes each breath.

If it gets very stressful I would take a break, reassure her, and try again later. Children are very much in tune with their parents' feelings so a positive attitude is essential. Always praise your daughter when she has used the inhaler.

It is important to record how she is responding to this medication, frequency and duration of symptom and rescue inhaler use, as this will determine what further treatment is needed.

> **Q:** My asthma is made worse by the house dust mite. Would an air purifier or ioniser be of help?

A: Dust mite allergy is a common problem for asthmatics in temperate climates. Since mites live and thrive in many sites throughout the house, they are difficult to reduce and impossible to eradicate.

House dust mites are too tiny to see. They eat the flakes of skin we constantly shed. House dust mites are in every home; it does not mean that our homes are dirty. They are found in furniture and carpets and especially in our beds. We breathe in their waste products, which may cause an allergic response in your airways. Signs of allergy to dust mites include: wheezing when you are vacuuming or dusting or when you enter a dusty room/house; asthma symptoms; sneezing or itchy eyes at night or first thing in the morning.

There are many preparations and devices available which claim to reduce or kill house dust mites or purify the air. Unfortunately, there is still no good objective evidence that they are effective in reducing asthma symptoms.

The following is a list of some simple measures recommended by the Asthma Society of Ireland to help:

- ✳ Use complete barrier covering systems on your mattress, duvet and pillow.
- ✳ If possible, remove all carpets and replace with hard flooring.
- ✳ Vacuum all areas frequently.

- ✳ Use a vacuum cleaner with a HEPA filter and good suction. Vacuum cleaners with HEPA filters are more effective at picking up the house dust mite and do not scatter dust.

- ✳ Damp dust all surfaces or use an attachment on your vacuum cleaner.

- ✳ Keep soft toys to a minimum and wash at 60 degrees Celsius on a weekly or fortnightly basis.

- ✳ Hot wash (at 60 degrees Celsius) sheets, duvets and pillow cases once a week.

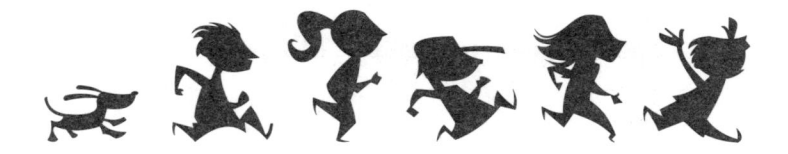

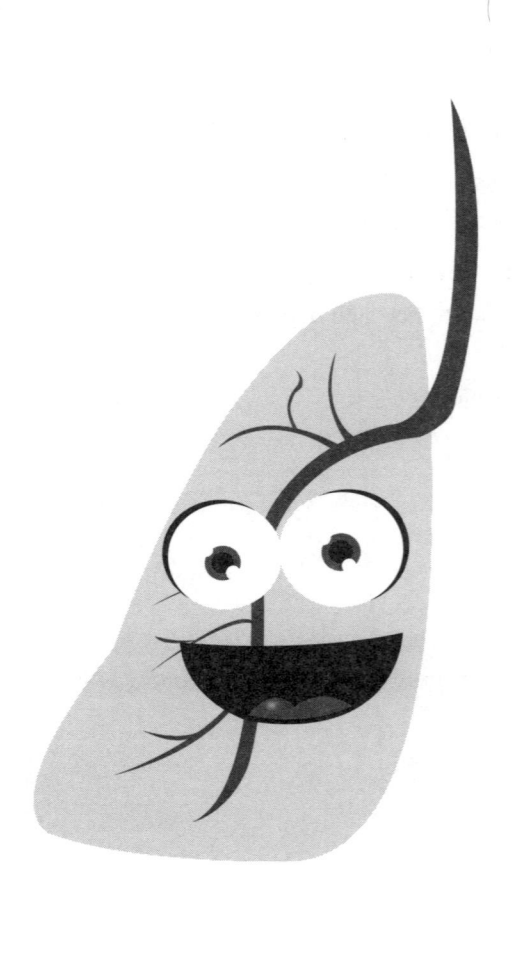

Further Sources of Information

- **Asthma Society of Ireland** (www.asthmasociety.ie)
- **European Federation of Asthma & Allergies** (www.efanet.org)
- **Global Initiative for Asthma** (www.ginasthma.com)
- **The Irish Anaphylaxis Campaign** (www.irishanaphylaxis.org)
- **Allergy Counts** (www.allergycounts.com)
- **Anaphylaxis Campaign** (www.anaphylaxis.org.uk)
- **Allergic rhinitis and its effect on asthma (ARIA)** (www.whiar.org)
- **Irish Eczema Society** (www.eczemaireland.org)
- **National Eczema Society** (www.eczema.org)
- **British Association of Dermatologists** (www.bad.org.uk)

* **Scottish Intercollegiate Network/British Society asthma guidelines**
  (www.sign.ac.uk/guidelines/fulltext/101/index.html)

* **Child asthma control test**
  (www.asthmacontrol.com/child.html)

* **American Academy of Allergy Asthma & Immunology** (www.aaaai.org)

* **Allergic rhinitis and its effect on asthma**
  (www.whiar.org/Documents&Resources.php)

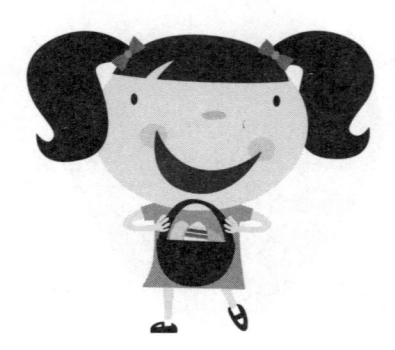

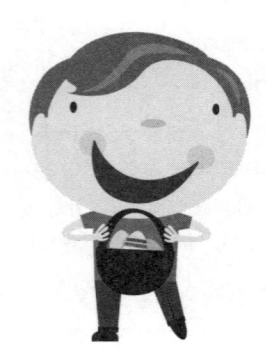

Glossary

Acute describes symptoms of rapid onset and short duration; opposite of chronic.

Adherence (also known as compliance) describes how compliant a patient is with their prescribed medication regime.

Adrenalin is a naturally occurring hormone produced by the adrenal gland. It increases heart rate, contracts blood vessels, dilates air passages and participates in the fight-or-flight response of the sympathetic nervous system. It has many medical uses, including the treatment of anaphylaxis, e.g. Anapen or Epipen.

Aspiration refers to the inhalation of foreign materials into the bronchial tree, usually oral or gastric contents (including food, saliva or nasal secretions).

Aerochamber is a small spacing device often used with a face mask to deliver inhaled medication to infants and toddlers.

Allergen is a non-parasitic substance capable of stimulating a type-I hypersensitivity reaction in atopic people.

Allergy is a disorder of the immune system which is a form of hypersensitivity. Allergic reactions occur to normally harmless environmental substances or foods, known as allergens.

Allergic rhinitis/Seasonal allergic rhinitis is an inflammatory condition of the lining of the nasal passages either related to a perennial allergen (e.g. dust mite), or seasonal allergen (e.g. grass pollen).

Allergic sensitisation is a reaction to a commonly occurring environmental or food substance identified using either skin or blood testing. Sensitisation does not indicate that there is disease.

Allergy tests There are two validated types of testing for immediate hypersensitivity: skin tests and blood tests. Skin allergy testing is a method for diagnosis of allergies that attempts to provoke a small, controlled allergic response. Results are available almost immediately. Specific IgE can be measured in the bloodstream by a RAST or CAP test. The sample is then forwarded to a laboratory to perform the assay. Results may take several days/weeks.

Alveoli are air sacs attached to the end of the bronchial tube, which permit the exchange of oxygen for carbon dioxide through very thin walled blood vessels called capillaries.

Anaphylaxis is an acute multi-system severe allergy reaction usually involving the skin, respiratory tract and circulation.

Antihistamine is a drug that blocks the receptor (H1) for the chemical histamine, which is released from mast cells and is involved in allergy inflammation, e.g. Citirizine (Zirtek®) and Loratidine (Clarityn®).

Antileukotriene (sometimes referred to as a leukast) is a drug that inhibits leukotrienes, which are fatty compounds produced by the immune system that cause inflammation in asthma and bronchitis, and constrict airways. Leukotriene inhibitors (or modifiers), such as montelukast, zafirlukast and zileuton, are used to treat those diseases. Leukotriene inhibitors are generally more variable in the clincial efficacy than corticosteroids, but have virtually no side effects, so they are often used to treat children.

Asthma attack A sudden worsening of asthma, an exacerbation of asthma or an asthma flare-up.

Atopic dermatitis (also known as eczema) is chronic inflammatory and itchy rash disorder which particularly affects the areas behind the knee and in the elbow creases.

Atopy A special or atopic syndrome; an allergic hypersensitivity affecting parts of the body not in direct contact with the allergen.

Babyhaler is a spacing device with a mask through which inhaled medications are taken.

Body Mass Index (BMI) is a measure of body weight based on a person's weight and height. Though it does not actually measure the percentage of body fat, it is used to estimate a healthy body weight based on a person's height.

Bronchi are a series of branching tube passages of airway in the respiratory tract that conduct air into the lungs. No gas exchange takes place in this part of the lungs.

Bronchioles are the first airway branches that no longer contain cartilage. They are branches of the bronchi. The bronchioles terminate by entering the circular sacs called alveoli.

Bronchiectasis is a disease state defined by localised, irreversible dilation of part of the broncial tree. It is classified as an obstructive lung disease, along with emphysema and cystic fibrosis. Involved bronchi are dilated, inflamed and easily collapsible, resulting in airflow obstruction and impaired clearance of secretions. Bronchiectasis is associated with a wide range of disorders, but it usually results from infections such as measles, whooping cough, staphylococcus and Klebsiella.

Bronchoconstriction is the constriction of the airways in the lung due to the tightening of surrounding smooth muscle with consequent coughing, wheezing, and shortness of breath.

Bronchial provocation test is a special form of breathing test that attempts to provoke asthma changes (using a variety of stimuli including drugs, exercise, cold air or low amounts of inspired carbon dioxide) in individuals who have normal pulmonary function. Typically, the test is considered positive when the FEV1 falls below 20 percent.

Bronchial hyper-reactivity or **hyper-responsiveness** is a key component of asthma, which describes the ease with which a stimulus provokes an asthmatic response on pulmonary function test using a bronchial provocation test.

Bronchodilator is a substance that widens the calibre of the bronchi and bronchioles, decreasing airway resistance and thereby facilitating airflow. Bronchodilators may be endogenous (originating naturally within the body), or they may be medications administered for the treatment of breathing difficulties.

Bronchomalacia is a condition of the airways where there is excessive collapsibility of the bronchi leading to impairment of airflow and mucociliary clearance. It may be misdiagnosed as asthma and is usually diagnosed by bronchoscopy.

Buteyko method or **Buteyko Breathing Technique** is a form of physcial therapy used for the treatment of asthma. The method takes its name from the late Ukrainian doctor Konstantin Pavlovich Buteyko, who first formulated its principles during the 1960s. The basic premise is that asthma can be effectively treated by altering an abnormal pattern of breathing condition called hyperventilation (rapid shallow breathing), which is the primary underlying problem. We now know that this is not the case. However, this method, in several small clinical trials, has been shown to safely reduce asthma symptoms and the need for rescue medication, as well as increasing quality of life scores. However, improvement takes time and commitment, requiring daily exercises over a period of weeks or months. At the core of the Buteyko method is a series of reduced-breathing exercises that focus on nasal-breathing, breath-holding and relaxation. Buteyko's theory was that asthmatics 'chronically overbreathe' and the exercises are designed to teach asthmatics to breathe less. The goal is to retrain breathing to a normal pattern, akin to certain forms of yoga.

CAMP study The Childhood Asthma Management Program was initially designed to evaluate whether continuous, long-term treatment (over a period of four to six years) with either an inhaled corticosteroid (budesonide) or an inhaled non-corticosteroid drug (nedocromil) safely produces an improvement in lung growth, as compared with treatment for symptoms only (with salbutamol and, if necessary, prednisolone, administered as needed). The primary outcome in the study was lung growth, as assessed by the change in forced expiratory volume in one second (FEV1, expressed as a percentage of the predicted value) after the administration of a bronchodilator. Secondary outcomes included the degree of airway responsiveness, morbidity, physical growth, and psychological development. The CAMP study has expanded into a long-term follow-up of the effects of asthma into early adulthood.

Chronic means to last a long time, the opposite to acute.

Cochrane Reviews is a database of systematic reviews and meta-analysis, which summarises and interprets the results of medical research. The Cochrane Library aims to make the results of well-conducted controlled trials readily available and is a key resource in evidence-based medicine.

Cohort study is a form of longitudinal study used in medicine, econometrics and ecology. It is an analysis of risk factors and follows a group of people who do not have the disease, using correlations to determine the absolute risk of subject contraction. It is one type of clinical study design. Cohort studies are largely about the life histories of its subjects, e.g. Tuscon or CAMP cohorts.

Controller Medications, also known as preventers, are drugs used on a daily basis for patients with asthma whose symptoms are not mild or episodic. These medications are used to prevent asthma symptoms. They are normally taken daily for many months or years.

Corticosteroids, also known as steroids or glucocorticosteroids, are synthetically-produced versions of naturally occurring glucocorticoids, which are produced at physiologic concentrations by the adrenal cortex. At higher doses, corticosteroids are potent anti-inflammatory drugs which act at many levels of the inflammatory process. They are used topically or locally in many inflammatory conditions.

Cytokines (Greek *cyto-*, cell; and *-kinos*, movement) are small cell-signalling protein molecules that are secreted by the glial cells of the nervous system and by numerous cells of the immune system and are a category of signalling molecules used extensively in intercellular communication. Cytokines can be classified as proteins, peptides, or glycoproteins; the term 'cytokine' encompasses a large and diverse family of regulators produced throughout the body by cells of diverse embryological origin. In asthma the relevant cytokines are mainly immunoregulatory.

Cystic fibrosis is the commonest inherited life-shortening condition of Caucasians. It is inherited in an autosomal recessive fashion. A multi-system disorder, the condition is caused by a defective chloride channel in the apical epithelia, which in the airway leads to poorly hydrated secretions that interfere with mucociliary clearance and lead to irreversible pulmonary damage and death from respiratory failure.

Differential diagnosis is a medical term which lists, in order of priority, the potential diseases responsible for a given set of symptoms and physical signs.

Desensitisation is a form of immunotherapy that involves administration of small doses of allergen in order to produce an IgG response, which eventually overrides the excessive IgE response seen in allergic disorders.

Dry Powder Inhaler is a device used to deliver tiny powder particles of medication to the lower airways, e.g. Turbohaler, Diskus accuhaler.

Dust mites (*Dermatophagoides pteronyssinus*) are microscopic insects that feed on organic detritus, such as flakes of shed human skin, and flourish in the stable environment of dwellings. House dust mites are a common cause of asthma and allergic symptoms worldwide. Some of the gut enzymes (notably proteases) that persist in their faecal matter can be strongly allergenic. The house dust mite survives in all climates, even at high altitude. House dust mites thrive in the indoor environment provided by homes, specifically in bedrooms and kitchens. Dust mites survive well in mattresses, carpets, furniture and bedding, with figures around 188 animals per gram of dust. Even in dry climates, house dust mites survive and reproduce easily in bedding (especially in pillows), deriving moisture from the humidity generated by human breathing, perspiration and saliva.

Eosinophils, usually called eosinophils (or, less commonly, *acidophils*), are white blood cells that are one of the immune system components responsible for combating multicellular parasites and certain infections in vertebrates. Along with mast cells, they also control mechanisms associated with allergy and asthma. They are granulocytes that develop during haematopoiesis in the bone marrow, before migrating into the blood.

Epidemiology is the study of factors affecting the health and illness of populations. It serves as the foundation of interventions made in the interest of public health and preventive medicine.

Expiration is the movement of air out of the bronchial tubes, through the airways, to the external environment during breathing. Exhaled air is rich in carbon dioxide, a waste product of cellular respiration.

Generic is the chemical name of a drug of which there may be many different brands, e.g. Salbutamol is the generic, Ventoilin® is the brand.

Genomic imprinting is a genetic phenomenon by which certain genes are expressed in a parent-of-origin-specific manner. It is an inheritance process independent of the classical Mendelian inheritance. Imprinted genes are expressed only from the allele inherited from the mother or the father.

Hypersensitivity (Type 1) or immediate hypersensitivity is one of four types of hypersensitvity reaction. It is closely associated with allergic disease. It is characterised by excessive activation of certain white blood cells called mast cells and basophils by a type of antibody known as IgE, resulting in an extreme inflammatory response. Common allergic reactions include eczema, hives, hay fever, asthma attacks, food allergies, and reactions to the venom of stinging insects such as wasps and bees.

Histamine is an organic nitrogen compound involved in local immune responses as well as regulating physiological function in the gut and acting as a neurotransmitter. Histamine triggers the inflammatory response. As part of an immune response to

foreign pathogens, histamine is produced by basophils and by mast cells found in nearby connective tissues. Histamine increases the permeability of the capillaries to white blood cells and other proteins, in order to allow them to engage foreign invaders in the infected tissues which cause vasodilation,
bronchoconstriction, bronchial smooth muscle contraction, separation of endothelial cells (responsible for hives), and pain and itching due to insect stings.

Hygiene hypothesis is a concept to explain the high prevalence of asthma and allergic disease in developed countries. It proposes that in the absence of infestations and significant early infection, a switch occurs in our immune system which facilitates the excess production of the allergy antibody IgE, rather than our normal protective antibody IG.

Immunoglobulins are proteins found in the blood, which are used by the immune system to identify and neutralise foreign objects, such as bacteria and viruses. They are typically made of basic structural units—each with two large heavy chains and two small light chains—to form, for example, monomers with one unit, dimers with two units or pentamers with five units. Antibodies are produced by a kind of white blood cell called a plasma cell. There are several different types of antibody heavy chains, and several different kinds of antibodies, which are grouped into different isotypes based on which heavy chain they possess. Five different antibody isotypes (A,D,E,M & G) are found in mammals, which perform different roles, and help direct the appropriate immune response for each different type of foreign object they encounter.

Immunoglobulin E (IgE) is a class of antibody that has only been found in mammals. It plays an important role in allergy, and is especially associated with Type-1 hypersensitivity. IgE has also been implicated in immune system responses to most parasitic worms like *Schistosoma mansoni, Trichinella spiralis*, and *Fasciola hepatic* and may be important during immune defense against certain protozoan parasites such as *Plasmodium falciparum*.

ISAAC is the International Study of Asthma and Allergies in Childhood. It is a unique worldwide epidemiological research programme established in 1991 to investigate asthma, rhinitis and eczema in children due to considerable concern that these conditions were increasing in western and developing countries.

Immunotherapy is the treatment of disease by inducing, enhancing, or suppressing an immune response. See desensitisation.

Inflammation is a component of the biological response of vascular tissues to harmful stimuli, such as infection, damaged cells, or irritants. Inflammation is a protective attempt by the organism to remove the injurious stimuli and to initiate the healing process.

Influenza, commonly referred to as the flu, is an infectious disease caused by viruses of the family *Orthomyxoviridae* (the influenza viruses), that affects birds, mammals and humans. The most common symptoms of the disease are chills, fever, sore throat, muscle pains, severe headache, coughing, weakness/fatigue and general discomfort.

Inspiration (also known as inhalation) is the movement of air from the external environment, through the airways, and into the alveoli.

Larynx, commonly called the voice box, is an organ in the neck of mammals involved in protecting the trachea and sound production.

Leukotrienes are fatty molecules of the immune system that contribute to inflammation in asthma and allergic rhinitis, synthesised by the 5-lipoxygenase pathway in leukocytes (especially mast cells), eosinophils, neutrophils, monocytes and basophils.

Mast cell (or mastocyte) is a resident cell of several types of tissues and contains many granules rich in histamine and heparin. Although best known for their role in allergy and anaphylaxis, mast cells play an important protective role as well, being intimately involved in wound healing and defence against germs.

Meta-analysis is when multiple individual studies that address the same question are combined the enable more powerful statistical inferences to be derived.

Metered-dose inhaler (MDI) is a device that delivers a specific amount of medication to the lungs, in the form of a short burst of aerosolised medicine that is inhaled by the patient.

Methacholine is a synthetic chemical that acts as a non-selective muscarinic receptor agonist in the parasympathetic nervous system. Its principal clinical use is to diagnose bronchial hyper-reactivity, which is the hallmark of asthma.

Mucosa (or mucus membrane) describes the cells that form the lining of cavities within organs that are exposed to the external environment.

Mucus describes secretions produced by mucosal cells.

Nasal polyps are polypoidal masses arising mainly from the mucous membranes of the nose and paranasal sinuses. They are overgrowths of the mucosa that frequently accompany allergic rhinitis. They are freely moveable and non-tender.

Nebuliser is a device which converts fluid into a fine mist to be delivered to the lungs.

Peak expiratory flow meter is a small, hand-held device used to monitor a person's ability to breathe out air. It measures the airflow through the bronchi and thus the degree of obstruction in the airways.

Phenotype is any observable characteristic of an organism that results from the expression of its gene, and the interaction between the gene and environmental factors.

Physical signs are findings detected by a clinician on examination, as part of a clinical evaluation.

Prevalence is a measure used in epidemiology and is defined as the total number of cases of a condition that exist in a given population at a certain time. It is used as an estimate of how common a condition is within a population.

Puberty is the process of physical changes by which a child's body becomes an adult body capable of reproduction.

Pulmonary function tests (also known as lung function tests) are tests that demonstrate how the lungs are working and can help to determine the type of lung disease. They are also useful for tracking disease over time and determine how patients respond to treatment.

Sensitisation refers to the finding of a specific IgE response (a positive allergy test) to an allergen, which under normal circumstances is harmless. Sensitisation does not necessarily mean illness or disease; many atopic individuals may be sensitised to allergens which cause them no harm or to which they are tolerant.

Sinuses (or paranasal sinuses) are air-filled spaces, communicating with the nasal cavity, within the bones of the skull and face.

Sinusitis refers to infection within the paranasal sinuses.

Spacer is a perspex container into which an aerosol-containing asthma treament is sprayed. Some have a mouthpiece, e.g. Volumatic; others have a face mask attached, e.g. Aerochamber.

Spirometry is a type of lung function test performed using a device which measures how much air moves in and out of the lungs.

Symptom is a complaint or feeling of illness noticed by a patient or their parent elicited by the doctor during the clinical evaluation.

Trachea is the windpipe or main breathing tube connecting the upper airway to the bronchial tubes.

Trigger is something that can bring on an asthma attack, e.g. head colds or exercise.

Urticaria (or hives) are a transient skin rash characterised by itchy, red, raised bumps. Hives are frequently, but not always, caused by allergic reactions.

Upper respiratory tract infections (URI or URTI) are illnesses caused by an acute infection that involves the upper respiratory tract (nose, sinuses, pharynx or larynx). By definition it does not affect the trachea, bronchi or lungs.

Vocal cord dysfunction (VCD) is a condition that affects the vocal cords and is characterised by full or partial vocal fold closure, which usually occurs during inhalation for short periods of time. However, the condition can occur during both inhalation and exhalation. VCD can produce an expiratory sound which may mimic asthma. The condition is diagnosed by laryngoscopy and treatment usually consists of speech and language therapy.

Volumatic is a type of spacer.

Viruses are small infectious agents that can replicate inside the living cells of organisms. Most viruses are too small to be seen directly with a microscope, e.g. rhinovirus, RS Virus and Influenza. Antibiotics are ineffective against these types of germ.

Viral upper respiratory infection is an infection which predominantly affects the upper respiratory tract.

Wheeze is to breathe with difficulty while making a whistling sound, which happens when the bronchial tubes have narrowed. The noise occurs mainly during exhalation.

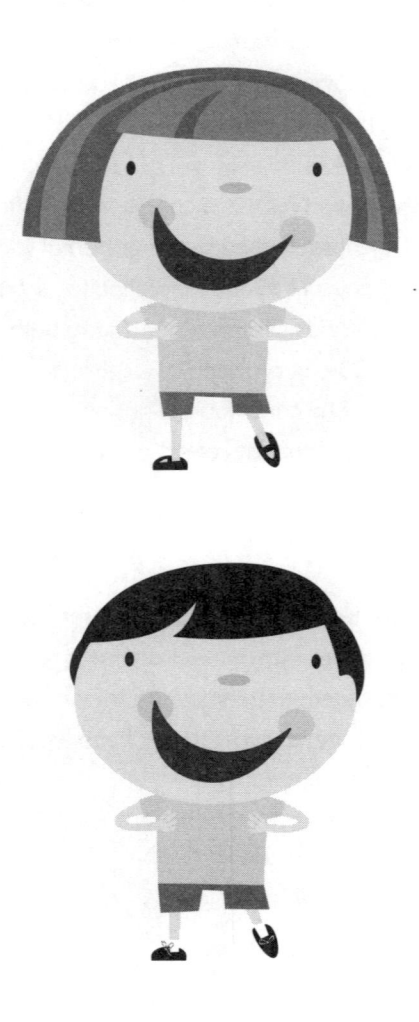